Critical Praise for the Bestselling
Dr. Mercola's Total Health Program

"Dr. Joseph Mercola is widely considered to be the world's top natural health physician practicing today, and his dietary program—presented in its entirety in *Dr. Mercola's Total Health Program*—has deservedly become the leading plan among those truly committed to losing weight permanently, preventing disease, looking and feel younger, and living longer. If you seek another fad diet, look elsewhere. If you seek a proven and permanent solution, do yourself a big favor and read Dr. Mercola's Total Health book as soon as possible."

> – John Gray, Ph.D., author of the blockbuster bestselling *Men Are From Mars, Women are From Venus* series of books

"Dr. Joseph Mercola is at the forefront of a health revolution that will change the face of our nation… This book, his most important written work yet, uses the wisdom gleaned from thousands of studies; more importantly, however, is that his program has actually succeeded in helping thousands of patients overcome seemingly "incurable" ailments… *Dr. Mercola's Total Health Program* is not a book to read once and put on your shelf to collect dust; instead, certainly for the recipes but also for the health and dietary insight in Part One and throughout, you'll find yourself referring back to it often as your trusted guide on the road to optimal health."

> – Jordan S. Rubin, N.M.D., Ph.D., Founder & Chairman of Garden of Life, author of the bestseller, *The Maker's Diet*

"Dr. Mercola is one of very few physicians who combine a very-long-term view of diet and human health with individualized diet recommendations. He's one of even fewer who help his patients improve their health and prevent disease by combining diet principles with attention to emotions and body energies. If you haven't read anything by Dr. Mercola before, you'll get excellent advice in *Dr. Mercola's Total Health Program*… You'll learn much, much more about getting well and staying well!"

> – Dr. Jonathan V. Wright, M.D., Medical Director of the Tahoma Clinic, Renton, Washington, author of *Natural Hormone Replacement for Women Over 45*

"I have been amazed that, as a 59 year-old "educated" male, I was so ignorant of many of the things promoted in the commercial media that are actually causes of health problems! I recently purchased *Dr. Mercola's Total Health Program* and to say it has changed my life would be an understatement. My wife says I look terrific, and I KNOW I feel better, have more energy than I had 10 years ago and my weight is now under control! Thanks, Dr. Mercola, you have made a difference in my life!"

– Rick McLellan, Land O Lakes, FL

"Just because you're thin doesn't mean you are healthy!! I have always been small in stature and size but health problems don't take this into consideration before entering your body. One year ago I was diagnosed stage three melanoma cancer. I didn't eat correctly nor did I take good care of my emotions. I have come through the cancer and to date have none remaining in my body. I owe a great deal of gratitude to Dr. Mercola for sharing so much of his knowledge, educating me on how to eat properly and how to take care of my emotions. I can tell such a difference in myself and so can people around me. I have read *Dr. Mercola's Total Health Program* and I never miss a newsletter. With these tools I feel like my life will be so much more healthy and rewarding. Thank you Dr. Mercola for sharing your wisdom so freely with people just like me who want to live a long prosperous life."

– Jewelie Weaver, Lancaster, CA

"*Dr. Mercola's Total Health Program* has dramatically changed my life. Before putting into practice these basic beginning principles, I was overweight, borderline diabetic and miserable with myself as well as having no energy. I began focusing on changing my behaviors as well as what I put into my body. In a short amount of time, I have lost 20 pounds and have gained amazing energy. I can finally play with my children longer and are continuing to see benefits that I didn't know were possible. I have always had trouble with sinus infections and colds and those have dramatically decreased in severity and frequency. I look forward to continued health improvements and weight stabilization as I continue implementing these life-changing steps. I recommend everyone find their true metabolic type and see what it can do for you."

– M. Roeder, Rambleridge, NE

"Mercola.com has been my number one resource for authentic integrative health advice. As a retired nurse and graduate of Capital University of Integrative Medicine my family and friends have counted on me to help them with nonpharmaceutical health matters. I have *Dr. Mercola's Total Health Program* which I have read and use religiously to help numerous people. Recently, on a visit to Kenya, I logged onto Mercola.com for information, and introduced another area of the world to the best e-newsletter ever written. Thanks Dr. Mercola. We need you."

– Jean Johnson, Dale City, VA

"I found out about *Dr. Mercola's Total Health Program* through my family doctor. He has a copy in his waiting room and follows Dr. Mercola's dietary guidelines. Since starting on the Total Health Program, my husband lost 25 lbs. in 4 months, and his cholesterol went down 80 points! I lost the weight I had gained during pregnancy a year earlier, plus another 10 lbs. This plan has also helped me tremendously with controlling the hypoglycemic blood sugar swings that I had when I was feasting on a white flour, high sugar diet all the time. The Mercola.com website has an amazing amount of information on getting and staying well using your body's own healing powers and proper nutrition."

– Lynette White, Ahwahnee, CA

"After purchasing *Dr. Mercola's Total Health Program*, I have dropped 40 pounds and am not constantly hungry as I was when I was eating grains and sugars. I own and operate a bakery, so it was very hard on me to have all the fresh baked goodies and not eat them. It is now much easier to pass on the goodies... they just taste too sweet! Thank you."

– Judy Beeman, Port Arkansas, TX

"Since ordering *Dr. Mercola's Total Health Program* I have started an exercise program and am careful about what I eat. I have particularly noticed a difference in my cravings for sugar. When I don't eat sugar, I don't crave sugar. I have lost a total of 12 pounds so far. It's amazing to discover the truth about nutrition and how to understand grocery labels. The information in this book is priceless!! I come from a very unhealthy family and Dr. Mercola's book has helped us tremendously!! If everyone would follow Dr. Mercola's advice on nutrition and exercise, our Nation would be a much healthier and wealthier place. I can't believe the difference in myself in such a short period of time. I look forward to each day and the opportunity to exercise and come closer to my goals of my new self."

– Lori Watson, Holdrege, NE

"*Dr. Mercola's Total Health Program* has changed my life. I have begun by incorporating two or three changes at a time. I thought I'd have to spend the rest of my life feeling deprived. NOT! About once every other week I read through it again, and learn something totally new, and begin to slowly include it in my lifestyle. I've been a health nut for over 20 years, and I thought I knew it all. Dr. Mercola has pleasantly educated me even more. Dr. Mercola, thank you from my heart."

– Vicki Worthington, San Antonio, TX

"I subscribed to Dr. Mercola's newsletter and was immediately hooked. I then purchased *Dr. Mercola's Total Health Program*. I was never what you would call fat but at the age of 49 had an extra 20 pounds that I wanted to get rid of. I did not go on a diet. I changed my thinking about food completely based on the aforementioned reading and not only lost the twenty pounds but have better skin tone, the energy of a 17 year old. I now sleep through the night and have rid my self of menopausal symptoms. My three grown daughters have started to take me seriously now when I talk to them about nutrition. I have independently verified a great deal of the information on Dr. Mercola's site and found him to be forthcoming, succinct, honest and resourceful. My thanks for the ongoing education."

– Harmony Boyer, Seattle, WA

DR. MERCOLA'S
TOTAL HEALTH PROGRAM

The Proven Plan to Prevent Disease and Premature Aging,
Optimize Weight and Live Longer!

by Dr. Joseph Mercola

with Brian Vaszily, Dr. Kendra Pearsall and Nancy Lee Bentley

Mercola.com
1443 West Schaumburg Road
Schaumburg, IL 60194

Dr. Mercola's Total Health Program:
The Proven Plan to Prevent Disease and Premature Aging,
Optimize Weight and Live Longer!

By Dr. Joseph Mercola, Brian Vaszily, Dr. Kendra Pearsall, and Nancy Lee Bentley

Publisher: Mercola.com
1443 West Schaumburg Road
Schaumburg, IL 60194

Publisher's Note: This book is intended as a reference volume only, not as a medical
manual. The ideas, procedures, and suggestions contained herein are not intended as a
substitute for consulting with your personal medical practitioner. Neither the publisher
nor the authors shall be liable or responsible for any loss or damage allegedly arising
from any information or suggestion in this book. Further, if you suspect that you have
a medical problem, we urge you to seek professional medical help.

ISBN 0-9705574-6-9

Design by Wendi S Rogers – www.sanguinedesign.com

First Edition, Seventh Printing. February 2005.

This book may be bulk ordered at special rates.
Contact customerservice@mercola.com or write to
Mercola.com, 1443 West Schaumburg Road, Schaumburg, IL 60194.

About the Authors

Dr. Joseph Mercola is the director of The Optimal Wellness Center in Chicago, one of the nation's leading natural health clinics, and the founder of Mercola.com, the world's most visited natural health website. He is also the author of the New York Times 2003 bestseller, *The No-Grain Diet*. As an Osteopathic Doctor, Dr. Mercola first trained in conventional medicine and later received extensive training in natural medicine. He has been in practice over two decades. Prior to The Optimal Wellness Center, he was Chairman of the Department of Family Practice at St. Alexius Hospital in Illinois for five years. He has been interviewed and profiled extensively for his health and dietary expertise, including ABC's World News Tonight, CNN, CBS, ABC, NBC, and Fox TV shows across the nation.

Brian Vaszily is the General Manager of Mercola.com and the Editorial Director of the Mercola newsletter with over 300,000 subscribers, the author of many articles, essays and other works published in magazines, newspapers and more nationwide, and the author of the critically-acclaimed novella about 9/11, *Beyond Stone and Steel*.

Dr. Kendra Pearsall is a Naturopathic Doctor at the Optimal Wellness Center who specializes in bariatric medicine and endocrinology (weight loss and hormones). Dr. Pearsall graduated in 2001 from Southwest College of Naturopathic Medicine, a four-year medical college in Tempe, AZ. Dr. Pearsall's greatest professional aspiration is to use her creativity to motivate the masses toward higher levels of physical, mental and spiritual well-being, a goal that she hopes to achieve in her next project of creating innovative weight loss and diabetes programs and educational seminars for the public.

Nancy Lee Bentley is a dynamic holistic health expert, chef, nutritional consultant, teacher, writer and speaker. This Cornell-educated food, nutrition, and communications professional, whose career spans over 25 years in the commercial and whole foods industry, foodservice, healthcare and media, has been called a pioneer in the fields of organic and natural foods, sustainable food systems and holistic health. Her work has appeared in national and regional publications, with recognition from Earl Nightingale, the USDA and 2000 Notable American Women, among others.

Table of Contents

Forward

by Jordan S. Rubin, N.M.D., Ph.D.,
Author of *The Maker's Diet*

Dr. Joseph Mercola is at the forefront of a health revolution that will change the face of our nation. With obesity, cancer, and heart disease at an all-time high and the incidence of digestive and immune-related disorders increasing by the moment, the time to change is now. I have known Dr. Mercola for over 4 years, and out of the thousands of physicians I speak to each year, he stands out as one of the most committed, driven, and insightful health practitioners today. Our mutual reverence for the timeless health truths set in motion at the creation of time has made us "kindred spirits" on a mission that is beyond even the scope of our imagination. His commitment to finding the highest quality solutions for his patients' health is second to none.

Always willing to step outside of the proverbial "box," Dr. Mercola is never satisfied with status quo; despite the nearly miraculous results he achieves with his patients on a daily basis, he is always looking to refine and improve his protocols. Through his groundbreaking website, Mercola.com, and the free e-newsletter available there—that, incidentally, is read by hundreds of thousands each week—Dr. Mercola gives all of us common sense truths, backed by history and science, that can make an immediate impact on our health if we take action.

This book, his most important written work yet, uses the wisdom gleaned from reading thousands of studies; more importantly, however, is that his program has actually succeeded in helping thousands of patients overcome seemingly "incurable" ailments. Through his book, Dr. Mercola leads us to a practical health plan that truly works.

Dr. Mercola's Total Health Program provides the reader with over 150 delicious, whole food recipes and a proven program for optimizing weight, energy, and health by eating the proper foods, and in the proper proportions according to one's specific biochemistry. The reader will learn about all the "right" and "wrong" foods, and how they can affect the quest for optimal health—physically and emotionally. By ignoring the notion of "politically correct nutrition," Dr. Mercola's new book provides us cutting-edge health information such as:

- Six essential steps to health and optimal weight that you need to know.
- Fourteen major ways sugar can cause serious health problems and how to avoid the risks.
- The high-sugar culprits (disguised by food manufacturers as "healthy") that are actually contributors to obesity and a variety of diseases in children and adults.
- The nine ways pasteurization destroys the health value of milk and what alternatives you have.
- Why sleep is one of the most important keys to health, and the 22 most effective ways to sleep well.

- Why red meat and eggs may actually be health foods and how to ensure you're consuming the right kind.
- The fat that can actually help you stay thin, improve your metabolism, and improve your immune system.

Those are just a few of the groundbreaking health secrets you will learn from reading and using this book. ***Dr. Mercola's Total Health Program*** is not a book to read once and put on your shelf to collect dust; instead, certainly for the recipes but also for the health and dietary insight in Part One and throughout, you'll find yourself referring back to it often as your trusted guide on the road to optimal health.

Let me be the first to congratulate you on making today the *first* day of the rest of your health. God Bless You!

- Jordan S. Rubin, N.M.D., Ph.D.
  Founder & Chairman, Garden of Life
  Author of the 2004 bestseller, *The Maker's Diet*

Forward
by Jonathan V. Wright, M.D.
Author of *Natural Hormone Replacement for Women Over 45*

Dr. Mercola is one of very few physicians who combine a very-long-term view of diet and human health with individualized diet recommendations. He's one of even fewer who help his patients improve their health and prevent disease by combining diet principles with attention to emotions and body energies. If you haven't read anything by Dr. Mercola before, you'll get excellent advice in this book, and I also recommend you visit his website, Mercola.com. You'll learn much, much more about getting well and staying well!

About that very-long-term view that Dr. Mercola takes: when I was a pre-medical student in the 1960s (according to my children, the "Dark Ages") I took the same courses in biology, chemistry, biochemistry, and physics that all the other pre-meds did. But I also majored in anthropology, because I thought that if I was going to try to take care of people's health, I'd best learn as much about us people as I possibly could.

I learned that the very first remains of any kind of people at all date back approximately 2 million years, and that remains of people who appear to be the same (with individual differences, of course) as we are date back *many thousands of years*. I also learned that, for all those years, what "we" (in this case, not you and me, but our ancestors) ate were various parts of various animals, fish, shellfish, the occasional egg stolen from a bird's nest, vegetables, roots, nuts, fruits and berries for a month or two a year, and insects (which is still done in parts of Australia). But until approximately 500 generations ago, when various groups slowly "invented" agriculture and domesticated animals, absolutely no one ate grains, and no one at all drank milk or ate any other dairy products! (Can you imagine a pre-historic cow holding still to be milked? Prehistoric cattle ran away from us humans as fast as they could!)

I took some history classes, too, and learned that only four to five hundred years ago refined sugar was as expensive as gold, so only kings and queens and the very wealthy could afford it, and only in very tiny quantities. Before that, no one had any at all! We learned that synthetic, artificial food chemicals, flavors, and preservatives were just invented in the 19th century, and margarine, too. Before then, no one ate any of these not-really-foods at all!

Meanwhile my biochemistry classes taught us that (with individual differences) your "modern" 21st century human biochemistry and mine "works" exactly the same as human biochemistry always has for the last *many thousands of years*. And it's very likely that human biochemistry has worked exactly the same (or incredibly close) for *many thousands of generations*.

What does a human biochemical system do? It manages the "stuff," the molecules and atoms of material reality, that helps keep us alive. (Of course material reality isn't everything: there's a whole universe of energy, there's psychology, spirituality—all of these are very important to your health and mine. But since the book you're about to read is almost entirely about diet, I'll stick with material reality for now.) And it just makes sense that if our personal biochemistries are exactly the same as human biochemistry has been for all that time, we'll stay healthier if we use the same materials (food and drink) to "fuel" that biochemistry that our ancestors have used for hundreds of thousands and millions of years. And if we can't duplicate those ancestral diets exactly, we should come as close as we possibly can.

Here is an (admittedly satirical) way of making the same point, from the first book I published (*Dr. Wright's Book of Nutritional Therapy*, 1979):

The hunter stalked his prey through the awakening forest. As the early rays of the sun filtered through the branches overhead, he moved noiselessly from tree to tree. Finally halting, he quickly but carefully fitted an arrow to his bowstring, aimed, and let fly. This time he hit his mark; he was glad, because he had not eaten since the previous day. He walked to where his arrow had fallen, carefully removed the chocolate-covered jelly doughnut, and walked away, eating his breakfast.

The four women had wandered far to find food for the midday meal. Finally the oldest, wise in the ways of their tribe, saw a familiar plant. She'd only seen it once as a girl, but had remembered. From it they gathered the cans of spaghetti and meatballs, and started home.

The children, thirsty again, ran to a tree they knew well. At this time of year, it provided the most delicious orange-flavored fruit drink, with 50% more vitamin C than the competing tree on the other side of their encampment...

Never happened, did it? And we shouldn't be eating that stuff, or anything else like it! And that's the very-long-term view that Dr. Mercola takes about diet and health.

But even though our general human biochemical patterns have been the same for all those years, we are all individuals with our own individual variations on the general human pattern. While individualization is what Dr. Mercola (and any good physician) does with each client he or she sees in person, individualization can't be done nearly as well by a book. But he makes a good start by helping you to apply the principles of "Metabolic Typing," which helps to group our individual biochemistries into several general patterns.

To conclude, if you're not feeling well and follow Dr. Mercola's advice in this book, your health will improve. If you have no health problems and don't want any, following his advice will keep most illness away.

And for his next book, I'll talk to Dr. Mercola about those elusive prehistoric cows.

– Jonathan V. Wright, M.D.
  Medical Director, Tahoma Clinic, Renton, Washington – www.tahoma-clinic.com
  Author (with Lane Lenard, Ph.D.) of *Why Stomach Acid Is Good For You* (2001),
  Maximize Your Vitality and Potency for Men Over 40 (1999), *Natural Hormone
  Replacement for Women Over 45* (1997)

Preface

This book took over twenty years to complete. When it finally came time for a title, I hesitated calling it a mere cookbook because that implies just another collection of recipes, and as you'll soon discover, it's kind of like calling Mt. Everest just another hill. A hill you forget, but Mt. Everest permanently transforms you. In the sense of how long you live, and even more so how well, this "cookbook" is a full dietary and lifestyle plan—no matter who you are or what your health condition is—that will significantly transform your life.

Yes, that may sound lofty, but my integrity is important to me, and I am committing here in words for you that I am certain of it. How can I be so sure? Let me start by telling you a story. A few months ago, I had my first consultation with a wonderful woman named Sally. She was 45 years old, stood 5'1", weighed 300 pounds, and suffered severe depression, diabetes, anxiety attacks, extensive fatigue, insomnia, and rheumatoid arthritis symptoms—for starters. She was on an astounding twenty-five different prescription medications via her previous physicians, and had already undergone six major surgeries in her life. With all of this conventional "healthcare," though, she was still and with increasing momentum heading downhill.

Sally became a patient at my clinic for the same reason many chronically ill patients do. She was desperately fed up with the false promises of the Band-Aid approach of conventional medicine, which was obviously doing nothing to address the underlying causes of her conditions, and had heard about my program's immense success through treating the true cause of health problems and teaching people to make necessary lifestyle changes. Sure enough, within just two months Sally stopped ten of her most dangerous (and unnecessary) prescriptions, she'd already lost ten pounds, and experienced a dramatic decrease of her depression, anxiety, insomnia and fatigue, so that these once debilitating issues were no longer noticeable. Again, this was within the first two months, and Sally's health continues to improve. So was it some magic pill or complicated surgery I administered? Of course not. It was the program you will find in this book. We determined her metabolic type, recommended the ideal foods for her type, administered the tools to help her overcome emotional barriers, and recommended the few choice supplements and the exercise you'll find in these pages. She stuck with it, and experienced those dramatic results in a period of time much shorter than she had even dared to imagine.

Sally is not an exception but the rule with my program. Primarily through the program in Part One of this book, upon which all of the recipes in Part Two are based, my clinical team and I have helped many hundreds of people at even more extreme stages of illness and obesity improve and recover—many of them cases that conventional healthcare providers considered "lost causes." Meanwhile, my program has literally helped tens of thousands of people at earlier stages of chronic disease, with weight issues, and with other health conditions recover their health. This is both through The Optimal Wellness Center, my clinic just outside Chicago which is now the largest natural health center in Illinois, and my free e-newsletter and website, Mercola.com, which is currently the most visited natural health site in the world.

I am of course proud to have helped so many people already, but more so I am honored, and I thank God everyday for letting me do so. Frankly, I'm often still also amazed with the overweight, diabetes and other chronic disease epidemics raging worldwide, the media spotlight has recently been very strong on my program for it's particularly high success rate at helping people with those conditions. But there are the thousands more—those who were experiencing milder conditions, such as fatigue or frequent headaches, those who want to improve their athletic performance, and those who simply had the foresight to seek to prevent disease in the first place—whose health has also been transformed for the better by the plan. The bottom line is, no matter who you are, this plan will help you, likely even more than you anticipate.

If you think it all sounds a bit too "miraculous," well, I really can't blame you. Every day we're bombarded by ridiculous claims from new diets, supplements, pills and programs promising you the sun, stars and eternity but often delivering nothing more than dust. It's understandable if you're skeptical. And so you do deserve to know how the plan and all the recipes created specifically for this book will truly improve your health and life. Which takes us right back to my opening point:

This book took over twenty years to complete. Not the physical writing of it, of course, but the book's most important aspect: the dietary and lifestyle plan it is founded on. Beginning in the late 1970s, when I was still in medical school, I had a strong notion that nothing was more essential to health and healing than proper diet. A few years later, as a young physician, I began what would become my life's passion and mission: to determine through committed investigations and practice the true "ideal diet" to help people prevent chronic disease and weight issues, and to reach their highest potential living a long life full of energy and free from pain. In the late 1980s through early 90s I experienced some major transformations of my own regarding my perception of the conventional healthcare system—namely, that its foundation was fatally flawed, as it was almost exclusively centered on treatments and mere patchwork, but not prevention and reliance on the intrinsic healing capacity God gave each and every one of us. This further motivated me as I recognized that people were confused about what the "right" diet was. They had major amounts of conflicting advice about fats and proper nutrition, and were intentionally being misled toward devastating food choices and perceptions of healthcare by the fast food and pharmaceutical industry that had much to gain in the way of money and power from doing so. People deserved the real answer, not information tainted by politics or greed, and I was committed to finding that answer.

The history of my dietary plan upon which the recipes in this book are based is filled with many breakthroughs obtained through my investigations and review of the medical literature and, even more so, my clinical experience with patients over the past two decades. But I've been asked in interviews many times to name the most important ones, those that profoundly shifted and expanded my understanding and, once I implemented them into patient's lives, improved their conditions most dramatically. In chronological order, I'd have to say these are the big three:

1) Your health, whether you have disease, weight issues, or decent health already, will improve dramatically if you eliminate, or vastly reduce, the amount of grains and sugars you consume.

2) Your emotional health is directly related to your physical health, and by using the emotional health tools discussed in these pages, you will greatly improve your ability to permanently optimize your weight, fight and prevent disease, and live longer.

3) You, like all people, have a unique biochemistry, or "metabolic type." And there are specific foods, at specific levels, that are most ideal for your type. Conversely, some foods that are generally considered "healthy" may not be as healthy for you as you think. One of the important keys this book will help provide is learning your metabolic type and major metabolic typing principles so that you can both vastly and rapidly increase your dietary success.

These "Big Three" are covered in detail for you in Part One of this book, as are all the other tenets of my dietary plan that you need to know in order to use the recipes in Part Two for their healing, preventative, weight loss, performance-enhancing and life-extending abilities. By the time you finish Part One, you will have a true total health plan customized to you in particular. The wonderful thing about the plan is that it's entirely designed around what's *naturally* right for your body, so sticking to it, you will find, will simply be following a diet that your body naturally gravitates toward. Eating according to your metabolic type is not the challenge you may fear it will be and you will be astounded by the results.

Part Two contains all the new recipes based on the dietary plan, including the required ingredients, detailed how-to-prepare information, yield, and nutritional values. What's more, most recipes are really several recipes in one, because you get detailed information on how to "fine-tune" the recipe to make it more appropriate for your metabolic type. You can cook from the recipes in Part Two even if you haven't read Part one yet, but you'll find the recipes, and your health, will greatly benefit by reading Part One and learning your metabolic type. Finally, because central tenets of my dietary program include low-to-no grains or added sugars, if you are diabetic or cannot tolerate gluten or grain products, you would obviously benefit from these recipes without even reading Part One—but don't make that mistake. Again, by reading Part One you'll learn how to improve your condition dramatically.

Which all leads me to some final words on how this "much-more-than-just-a-cookbook" will help you transform your life and health. Because it is a major compilation of my twenty-plus years of developing a comprehensive dietary and lifestyle plan that will help you overcome and prevent disease and illness, increase your energy, optimize weight permanently, remain young-looking, live longer and better, and frankly, enjoy many truly delicious meals along the way, my top requirement was to find the premier team to pull it all together for you, and that requirement was definitely fulfilled:

Brian Vaszily is the general manager and editorial director of my website, Mercola.com, and my free health e-newsletter. He has been central to improving the quality and scope of the content, and to making it engaging to a wide audience. I regularly seek his counsel as I strive to improve the site and its mission and he has been invaluable in taking our efforts several giant leaps higher. I am delighted that he was able to devote his exceptional literary, editorial and management talents to help create this awesome resource to improve your health.

Dr. Kendra Pearsall is a Naturopathic Doctor at my clinic, The Optimal Wellness Center—and my partner. Dr. Pearsall specializes in weight loss and endocrine (hormone) problems. Her medical, culinary, and literary talents and her faithful love and support were instrumental in bringing this cookbook to fruition.

Finally, Nancy Lee Bentley is a professionally trained chef with a background in metabolic typing, nutrition and whole health principles who has been following my dietary program for some time. You will find the original recipes she has created here are utterly delicious, easy to prepare, highly nutritious, and right in line with my Total Health program.

In summary, if you're already familiar with my dietary and lifestyle plan, whether through my free health e-newsletter at Mercola.com or as a patient of The Optimal Wellness Center, you've made a wise choice—this is the book that finally "pulls it all together" in Part One while providing, in Part Two, delicious and healthy meals and snacks for every day of the year no matter what your condition or type. Furthermore, if you discovered this book because you were searching for low-carb, low-calorie, low-sugar, grain-free recipes that were excellent for weight loss and diabetes, it will provide you all that. But if you adhere to the principles that surround the recipes, you will discover a few special bonuses such as increased energy and focus, the ability for your body to fight and prevent illness and disease, a more youthful appearance, far less reliance on the healthcare system, and a longer and more fulfilling life.

With all that in mind, bon appétit!

Introduction: Why the Mercola Total Health Dietary Program?

You've heard it before but it bears repeating: nothing in life is more precious than your health. If you take care of your body not only do you prevent disease and illness and prolong your life, but you also vastly improve the quality of your life. You increase your daily energy, creativity, attention span and mental focus, allowing you to achieve more in the pursuit of whatever matters to you, such as family, career, athletics and hobbies. Your emotions are also elevated, so your self-esteem and outlook on life end up where they've always belonged: very positive. And you're not just considered attractive to others for your fit body and glowing appearance, but indeed magnetic because of the confidence, energy, upbeat attitude and overall life you exude.

My dietary program is proven to help you achieve all of these benefits. Through my health clinic, The Optimal Wellness Center, and through my website, Mercola.com—now the world's most visited natural health website with many tens of thousands of pages of useful free health information—this program has helped many thousands of people improve and recover from chronic disease and other illnesses, optimize their weight, and increase their physical, mental and emotional performance.

The program, and all the recipes you'll find in this book that follow the program, is based on this one essential principle: the type and quality of the food you eat has a profound influence on your health. It only takes common sense to understand that what you put into your body several times a day, every day, will have far more impact on your well-being than anything else you do. Yet over two-thirds of Americans are now overweight, with one-third at the even more dangerous level of clinical obesity, and countries such as Australia, Canada, and Britain are experiencing similar epidemic levels. Consequentially, we're also experiencing widespread levels of chronic disease such as diabetes, heart disease, and cancer that are directly associated with obesity and other diet-related causes. The fact that the type and quality of food you eat has a profound influence on your health may therefore sound like common sense, but something is misdirecting the majority of us far away from such common sense. This misdirection, and the failure of those who are aware of it to do anything about it, is costing many people their lives.

In your hands, though, you hold a real solution. No matter where you are starting from today—perhaps you have a weight problem, diabetes, high cholesterol, or some other health condition, or perhaps you are reasonably healthy—the recipes in this book, and the insight of the dietary program and metabolic typing that surround them, will help you achieve your health goals. You can optimize your weight, improve or even eliminate your health challenges, prevent new ones, and achieve all the benefits mentioned at the start of this chapter if you commit yourself to it. And therein lies the key—commitment.

Like anything else of true worth in this life, achieving real health through this book is ultimately your decision. The information and recipes for healthy living are all provided for you here, but only you can choose to first commit yourself to the program. This deserves your careful consideration, as it is not uncommon to hear people "wish" that they were healthier, had more energy, or could permanently lose weight, but in the next breath complain that taking the real steps toward doing so is "too costly" or "too time-consuming." Some of these people will then slump into their couches to watch TV for hours everyday, or they'll waste thousands of dollars per year on junk food, soft drinks, and other non-food stuff that merely satisfies an immediate urge. How is it that spending so much time and resources on these pursuits and products is more important than devoting them to health? It's really a matter of getting priorities straight, of remembering that you've just got this one life to live. To drive the point home, try this one question test:

Of these five things, which would you least want to have destroyed or eliminated:

1) Your car
2) Your TV
3) Your house
4) Your job
5) Your body

If you answered number 5, then you'll realize that a central priority in your life should be dedicated to ensuring that your body isn't destroyed or eliminated prematurely. (And if you answered anything besides number 5, turn immediately to the "Overcoming Emotional Barriers" chapter of this book.) While the recipes in this book have been created to be as quick and easy as possible, you should still recognize that they are not as quick and easy as unwrapping a Snicker's bar, nor are they as cheap. While you'll find that the dietary plan, lifestyle habits, and emotional tools covered in this book will make succeeding on this diet far simpler than you're anticipating right now, it still is not as simple as grabbing a Big Mac at McDonald's drive-up window. But the results in all aspects of your life will be infinitely more rewarding. It all starts with your choosing.

You can choose to keep wishing you were thinner, healthier, and younger looking but not take the steps to actually improve your health. Or you can choose to make achieving optimal health a true priority in your life, and dedicate yourself to achieving it through the proven advice, recipes, and resources this book offers. Read on if your health and life are worth that effort.

PART ONE

DR. MERCOLA'S TOTAL HEALTH PROGRAM

1: The Six Mercola Essentials

Congratulations! You've taken a crucial step on your journey to optimal health and weight by choosing to commit yourself to it. You may not recognize it so much now, but in just a few weeks, and then again in a few months, and then for the rest of your life, when you are living the wonderful health benefits this book will provide, you'll look back fondly on this decision as one of the major turning points of your life.

So let's start with the "Mercola Essentials," which are the basis of my dietary program, every recipe in this book, and your healthy life:

1) No matter what your health challenge is, you should eliminate or at least significantly reduce the sugars and grains, particularly the processed forms, in your diet, as you'll find out in the next chapter.

2) Despite what some of the fad diets out there have insisted, you need carbohydrates, protein, and fat in your diet. None of these are evil as some "experts" have made them out to be. The key is, first, understanding and choosing only the healthy type of each of these, which you will learn in Chapter 3 and 4, and second, consuming the right amount of carbohydrates, protein, and fat for your personal metabolic type, which you'll learn in Chapter 5.

3) You have a unique biochemistry, or metabolic type, and certain types of "nutritious" food are healthier for your metabolic type, while other types of "nutritious" food are actually less so. You must know your metabolic type if you truly want to optimize your health and fitness; Chapter 5 of this book provides you the means to do so, including the crucial concept of "listening to your body" and fine-tuning your diet accordingly. Part Two then provides further guidance on how to alter the recipes, and guide your eating toward your metabolic type.

4) Your emotional and mental well-being is directly tied to your physical health and your dietary success. Negative emotions such as cravings and addictions, low self-esteem, and past traumas will impact your ability to overcome disease and overweight/obesity issues, but there are solutions provided in Chapter 6 that will help you overcome these emotional obstacles.

5) You will not need to consume a shopping bag full of supplements because the healthy recipes and foods recommended in this book will typically provide you with most of the

nutrients you will need. The only exceptions are: A) the few supplements that nearly everyone needs such as fish oil with omega-3, as detailed for you in Chapter 7, and B) specific supplementation for those with special health challenges.

6)   Making certain other lifestyle choices are essential to your health success. This includes drinking plenty of pure water, getting proper sleep, exercising, and learning how to bypass the influences of institutions fostering the overweight and chronic disease epidemics for their own profit and power. You'll learn about all these in Chapter 7, as well.

As you are reading this book, there are two important points to keep in mind. First, it is crucial that you avoid becoming overwhelmed with all of the useful information or attempt to bite off more than you can chew. Some people, when they encounter all the dietary and lifestyle changes they should make toward optimal health and weight, become discouraged because they believe they have to make them *all* happen at one time. Others become over-motivated and *try* to make them all happen at one time. Both frequently lead to failure. The key with all the insight offered in this book—and adopting positive changes in any aspect of your life—is to implement it in manageable bites. That means establishing a plan for yourself over time, and implementing the changes in phases into your life. Chapter 8, "Pulling It All Together," will help you in this regard by providing a simple approach and key reminders you can use to prioritize and build your "manageable bites" plan.

Second, you will notice that the recipes in the cookbook include a wide range of foods. While many of these foods can generally be found in your local grocery or health food store, the cookbook includes specific brands of food items recommended for their superior health value. A key point to remember is food quality is dramatically different depending on the source. For example, one source of salmon, such as the Vital Choice brand that we offer through Mercola.com, is from the pure waters of the Alaskan wilderness. We have had the salmon laboratory tested and it is certifiably free of any harmful toxins. Meanwhile, though, the vast majority of salmon found in supermarkets is contaminated with either mercury or PCB's and is quite unhealthy for you. Choosing *quality* foods and health products can make all the difference in the world to your health and well-being.

Because this quality is essential, on my website and in my twice-weekly newsletters I have always made it a point to research and recommend what I have found to be the highest quality food and health products. In this book, I provide you the same detailed insight on the right *types* of foods. With most of the foods I recommend, such as vegetables or nuts, you'll be able to find them in virtually any grocery or health food store. With others, particularly the right *types* of fish, beef and other meat, you are not likely to find these in a typical grocery store. I encourage you to first check your local health food store for these specific foods with my recommended guidelines. Locally owned health food stores are a national treasure well deserving of your business, and they are usually eager to listen to your input on the goods they should carry. However, if you can't find them elsewhere, or if time is an issue for you, you can easily access the "Recommended Products" section on Mercola.com to learn how to obtain these products.

2: The Dangers of Grains and Sugars

If you made no other adjustments to your diet but eliminating or vastly reducing grains and sugars it is likely your health would rapidly improve and within days you'd start losing weight. Within weeks you'd have a very noticeable improvement in both areas. Within months, in addition to the dramatic health and weight improvement, you'd also be experiencing a tremendous increase in your energy, mental acuity, and positive focus. Continue with the program beyond that and you will significantly extend the amount of time you spend on this planet.

No matter what your health condition or metabolic type, you are strongly advised to eliminate or restrict your grain and sugar intake, particularly processed grains and sugars. Eliminating grains is especially necessary for those who are Protein Metabolic Types. Carbohydrate and Mixed Types can get by with consuming a limited amount of grains. In all cases, any grains you do consume should be *whole* grains (95% of the grains consumed in the U.S. are processed, which strips them of what limited nutritional value they do have). Those with celiac disease and gluten-sensitivities have an obvious additional need to avoid grains, particularly gluten which is found in wheat, spelt, rye, barley, and oats. For those with diabetes and other signs of elevated insulin such as obesity, high blood pressure or high cholesterol, it is crucial to eliminate grains and sugars.

Avoiding grains and sugars has been popularized by the recent low-carbohydrate dieting rage. Although low-carb dieting is effective for weight loss, the low-carb approach misses the fact that you need carbohydrates in your diet, to varying levels depending on your metabolic type. Every recipe in this book has been created around the principle that grains and sugars should be eliminated or severely restricted, and the processed forms of both in particular. There are good carbohydrates that should compose most of your carbohydrate intake, and they are found mostly in high fiber vegetables that grow above the ground. Your body prefers these complex carbohydrates because they slow the release of simple carbohydrates like glucose and decrease your insulin levels. Insulin is the fat-building hormone in the body; therefore, increases in insulin cause weight gain. On the other hand, there are "troublesome" carbohydrates that you need to reduce or eliminate from your diet, and they are found in grains, sugars and sugary foods, as well as starchy vegetables like potatoes. These carbohydrates will increase your insulin levels and tend to promote weight gain and illness.

With that important point in mind, let's take a look at some basic human physiology so you can begin to understand why grains and sugars should be avoided.

You are What They Ate

For over five hundred generations, humans have existed primarily on a diet of wild animals and vegetation. It was only with the advent of agriculture a mere 6,000 years ago—an extraordinarily small period in evolutionary time—that humans began ingesting large amounts of sugar and starch in the form of grains and potatoes in their diets. Indeed, nearly all of our genes were set before the advent of agriculture; so, in biological terms, our bodies are still those of hunter-gatherers.

While the shift to agriculture produced other indisputable gains for man, societies where the transition from a primarily meat/vegetation diet to one high in grains show a reduced lifespan and stature, increases in infant mortality and infectious disease, and higher nutritional deficiencies. Keep in mind that these ancient societies used entirely unrefined and organic grains. Today over 90% of grains are highly processed, making the negative consequences of grains far worse.

The physiology of contemporary humans has not changed much from our distant ancestors, and our bodies have never adapted to the excessive amount of carbohydrates from grains and sweets in our present-day diet. In fact, in a nation whose diet is still largely based on the severely misguided USDA Food Pyramid, which recommends an atrocious 6–11 servings of breads, cereals, rice and pasta per day, this surplus of insulin-spiking carbohydrates is the main reason for the overweight epidemic and the scourge of related chronic diseases like diabetes.

It is primarily your body's response to the overindulgence of grain and sugars, not your intake of fat, which makes you fat. Consuming sugar also impairs your white blood cell function and thereby decreases your body's immune system, making you more vulnerable to disease. Your body has a limited capacity to *store* carbohydrates, but it can easily convert those excess carbohydrates, via insulin, into body fat, which means the more excess carbohydrates, the more body fat. When a government recommends that its population consume 6–11 servings of grains per day, plus four servings of fruit (which is high in simple sugars), an overweight epidemic is the logical and inevitable result.

The fact is that any meal or snack high in carbohydrates from grains or sweets generates a rapid rise in blood glucose. To adjust for this rise, your pancreas secretes the hormone insulin into the bloodstream, which lowers your blood sugar. Insulin is essentially a storage hormone, developed over millions of years to help you store the excess calories from carbohydrates in the form of fat in the case of famine. Throughout most of our biological history, and certainly in many areas of the world today, there were frequent periods of mass starvation caused by droughts and other natural occurrences that depleted the availability of vegetation (containing the complex carbohydrates that are the carbs you should eat) and therefore the game animals that relied on this vegetation. The body gradually developed defenses against this starvation so it could convert any excess carbohydrates to fat so it could use its fat stores for energy over time. You are, in other words, walking around in a body well designed to pull you through potential starvation. The problem is, we live in a time and a place with the extreme opposite situation—we don't experience times of famine and instead we have an overabundance of grains, starches and sweets, and food companies are marketing them endlessly to us.

To make matters even worse, high insulin levels also lower two other important hormones—glucagon and growth hormone—that are responsible for *burning* fat and sugar and promoting muscle development. In other words, insulin produced from consuming excess carbohydrates found in grains and sugars promotes fat, and then wards off your body's ability to lose that fat and build muscle!

Additionally, insulin also *causes* hunger, and it's usually a hunger for sweets. As blood sugar increases following a carbohydrate meal, insulin is secreted to lower the blood sugar. The lowered blood sugar results in hunger, often only a couple of hours or less after the meal. If ignored long enough, the hunger turns into feeling ravenous, shaky, moody and ready to "crash" as a result of hypoglycemia or low blood sugars. In order to raise your blood sugars, your body will naturally crave high sugar foods like sweets or grains, which leads to a vicious roller coaster ride of high and low blood sugars. You progressively convert to a sugar and grain addict and this causes you to become increasingly fatter, fatigued, depressed and sick.

But now back to the good news. You have this book, and it provides you with a practical solution. By eating according to your unique and specific biochemistry, you'll find the craving for these unhealthy but tempting foods disappears. If there are any emotional barriers you encounter when making the transition, you'll learn in Chapter 6 about a powerful psychological technique that is profoundly impressive in overcoming psychological resistance. Furthermore, you will have all the healthy recipes to put your insight into action for every day of the year.

Beware the Unfamiliar Grain, Corn

Most people can easily name the common grains such as rice, wheat, oats, barley, and rye, but forget that corn also belongs in that category, as they perceive corn to be a vegetable.

Corn is a grain, and it has all the negative health impacts of a grain. According to recent research, the demise of certain Native American Tribes in earlier centuries can be mainly attributed to corn. Their eating patterns shifted away from the primarily meat and vegetation diet of a hunter-gatherer society to a homogenous diet based almost entirely on corn with the arrival of the Spanish. The research shows that the bones of the Native Americans during and after this transition show much higher evidence of anemia, dental cavities, osteoarthritis, infections and other health issues than those who lived prior to this transition.

Corn is relatively high in sugar, which is one of the main reasons it's America's number one crop, consuming over 80 million acres of U.S. land and sneaking its way into an endless array of food (and other) products. In its unprocessed or "whole" state, corn offers negligible health benefits at best; sweet corn, for instance, contains vitamin C. However, you are far better off avoiding the corn's negative health impacts on your health and obtaining higher quantities of vitamin C and many other antioxidants from real vegetables such as broccoli and asparagus.

You are best served by avoiding corn in its processed state. Food with labels containing corn derivatives such as corn syrup, fructose, high fructose corn syrup, corn oil, cornmeal, cornstarch, dextrose, monosodium glutamate, xanthan gum, and maltodextrin, have no place in your grocery cart. Corn sweeteners are actually now the most widely produced of all sweeteners, accounting for 55% of sweeteners on the market. This is primarily high fructose corn syrup, which is the dominant ingredient in soft drinks, fruit drinks, cookies, candies and other popular grocery store items. Consumption of high-fructose corn syrup increased from zero in 1966 to a whopping 62.6 pounds per person in 2001, and is a key culprit in the diabetes and overweight epidemic.

There is one more "hiding place" for corn that you must be aware of: in your beef. Most of the beef you'll find in grocery stores, and virtually all the beef used in fast food and other restaurants, is from cattle that were force-fed diets high in corn.

There are two more factors you should know about corn. First, corn is only second to soybeans as the most genetically modified (GMO) crop in the U.S. GMOs, which were first introduced in 1995, are a potential disaster waiting to happen, as no studies have been done with humans to show what happens when genetically modified foods are consumed. The Food and Drug Administration (FDA) has assumed that these modified foods are equivalent to the original foods, and therefore, does not require any studies to have them approved. This is despite the fact that: 1) this technology has never before existed in the history of the world, and 2) the United State's track record on genetically engineered safety is terrible.

Second, as you can read in detail in Doug Kaufmann and Dr. David Holland's book, *Infectious Diabetes*, corn is one of the foods highest in mycotoxins (wheat and several other grains are high as well), which are toxins from fungus that can lead to cancer, heart disease, diabetes and a wide host of other serious diseases.

Nevertheless, there is hope! One of the most profoundly important changes you can make immediately in your diet is to switch to consuming healthy meat. Atop this list is choosing nutritious and safe alternatives to corn-fed beef, such as grass-fed beef or grass-fed bison, which are discussed in detail in Chapter 4 and used in some of the recipes in this book.

Sugar, The Nemesis To Optimal Health

Most people are addicted to sugar, and along with grain addiction, the over-consumption of added sugars—whether they are high-fructose corn syrup, fructose, glucose, dextrose, or the sucrose from sugarcane and sugar beets—is one of the major health problems facing our nation today.

For just a partial idea of the ill health effects of excess sugar consumption, consider that sugar has been cited as a contributing factor to:

- Overweight and obesity
- Immune system suppression, inviting infection and disease
- Premature aging
- Cancer of the breast, ovaries, prostate, and rectum
- Decreased absorption of calcium and magnesium
- Diabetes
- Fatigue
- Decreased energy and reduced ability to build muscle
- Heart disease
- Crohn's disease and ulcerative colitis
- Osteoporosis
- Yeast infections
- Depression
- Dental decay and gum disease

Sugars are simple carbohydrates processed by the body in the same manner as grains. That is, any excess sugars in the body are converted by insulin into fat—and just like grains, we're consuming an enormous surfeit of sugar. In the past two decades in the U.S., sugar consumption has increased by over 30%. In fact, the average per-person sugar intake is now 175 pounds per year! That's 300,000 calories per year, or 800 calories per day, from sugar! This is asking for serious health trouble even by the ill-advised USDA standards, which states that the average American, who should be consuming about 2,000 calories per day, can eat up to 10 teaspoons of added sugars per day. The average American is consuming well over 3000 calories per day, including over 20 teaspoons of added sugars.

The majority of these added sugars are coming from soft drinks, which the average American drinks an estimated 56 gallons of each year. That's an average of 600 cans of soda pop per year *each!* Just one can of this soda has about 10 teaspoons of sugar and 150 calories, along with 30 to 55 mg of caffeine. Soda also contains harmful additives including phosphoric acid, which can interfere with the body's ability to use calcium, leading to osteoporosis or softening of the teeth and bones. Phosphoric acid also neutralizes the hydrochloric acid in your stomach, which can interfere with digestion, making it difficult to absorb nutrients. Eliminating soft drinks from the American diet—a distant but noble dream—would alone vastly reduce the rate of obesity and add years to our average lifespan.

Moreover, there are high-sugar culprits disguised as "healthy" by food marketers such as: "fruit drinks," "fruit beverages" and "fruit punch," such as Snapple, which contain anywhere from 1% to 40% of fruit juice but which all contain loads of sugar, usually high-fructose corn syrup.

But even the sugars in 100% real fruit juice can quickly add up: real fruit juice, whether store-bought or freshly squeezed, has about eight full teaspoons of sugar per eight-ounce glass. This sugar is typically a fruit sugar called fructose, which is every bit as dangerous as the regular table sugar sucrose since it will also cause a major increase in insulin levels.

This doesn't mean that you should avoid fruit, just fruit juice. When the fruit is intact and whole, its fiber will moderate the release of fructose and secondarily insulin into your bloodstream. However, if you are overweight, have high blood pressure or high blood sugar levels, you would be wise to avoid most fruits and just stick with vegetable carbohydrates until you have these problems under control. This is especially true if you are a Protein Metabolic Type. Carbohydrate types are generally better designed to handle the carbohydrates in fruits, especially citrus fruits.

On a different note, sugar substitutes such as saccharin (Sweet-N-Low), sucralose (Splenda) and aspartame (Equal and Nutrasweet) should be avoided. Their negative health effects can easily exceed the sugars they are replacing. Some scientists, for instance, believe aspartame might cause altered brain function and behavior changes. The FDA has also been inundated with consumer complaints about aspartame, including fibromyalgia symptoms, multiple sclerosis symptoms, dizziness, headaches, and menstrual problems. You can use the search engine on my site for further details on aspartame and its brand names like Nutrasweet.

You should also avoid the latest sugar substitute rage, sucralose. First of all, few human studies have been published on the safety of sucralose. Second, in animal research studies, sucralose was shown to cause a decrease in the size of thymus glands, to cause liver and kidney enlargement, reduce growth rate, decrease red blood cell count, and decrease placenta and fetal body weights—

and this is only a partial list. Sucralose also has the potential to contaminate your body with pesticides, heavy metals such as lead, arsenic, and more, as it has been found to contain small amounts of these dangerous substances. Finally, if you are trying to lower your weight, there is no clear evidence that sucralose—or any artificial sweetener—is even useful in weight reduction. In fact, there is evidence that these substances may actually *stimulate* your appetite.

For many people, sugar is an authentic addiction, akin to cigarette dependency. And it is affecting their health as severely as cigarettes would, if not more so. The real solution is not to keep hunting for ways to "safely" maintain the addiction, such as artificial sweeteners, which are kind of like the equivalent of "Light" and "Ultra Light" cigarettes—that is, equally as devastating to your body. The solution is to overcome the addiction. Fortunately, you'll find that by adopting this dietary plan, including eating the foods meant for your metabolic type and utilizing the tools to overcome emotional barriers described later in this book, you won't have to "fight" the craving, because it will naturally disappear. This has been the case for thousands before you, and if you stick to the principles in this book, it will be the case with you.

3: Plant-Based Foods: Mercola's Guide to the Healthiest

Mark Twain, when warned about the potential known health effects of smoking in his day, replied, "Quitting smoking may indeed add ten years to my life, but then that's ten years without a cigarette." This is the same excuse that many people use for not abandoning baked goods, breakfast cereals, popcorn, fried foods, sweets, soft drinks and other deadly foods: "Well I know it's bad for me and it's probably shortening my life, but it tastes so good and so it's making the life I am living so much better."

What Twain might not have known about cigarettes, and what the average person may not be aware of with eating junk food, is that it is not only likely to cause disease and shorten their life, but it is decreasing their quality of life by decreasing their energy, mental focus, and happiness. That is, for that brief "hit" of, say, Coca-Cola, toasted bagels, or French fries—just as with the brief hit of nicotine—they are giving up both their quality of life right now and the length of their life later. If you often feel more tired than you should, or experience "brain fogginess" where it's hard to focus, or you often feel down if not downright depressed, eating unhealthy food could be a primary culprit. Are those states really worth a bag of potato chips or pretzels?

Some of you may have an underlying fear that by converting to the truly healthy diet offered here, you will never again experience great-tasting food and it will instead be like chewing on tree bark. However, you'll quickly discover once you start trying the recipes in this book that they are delicious as well as nutritious. In fact, by eating according to your metabolic type, you will feel so much better that you will want to continue to eat the natural foods that your body is designed for. Nevertheless, if you still do experience cravings for unhealthy foods like sugar or grains after you begin selecting foods according to your metabolic type, you will have the emotional tools in Chapter 6 to overcome these barriers.

Eat Your Veggies!

There is no food group that is denser with vitamins, minerals, antioxidants, and flavonoids than the vegetable group. This is particularly true for the vegetables that grow above the ground. Vegetables provide the good carbohydrates you need, and much more. Those who are Protein Metabolic Types should ideally get most of their carbs from vegetables, with virtually none from grain or sugar-added foods. Those who are Carb Types should also ideally get most of their carbs from vegetables—and they need more carbs in total, but can do well getting about 15% of their carbs from healthy, *whole* grains if they choose. Mixed Types, as the name implies, fall in the middle of these two.

The glycemic index is a measure of how quickly after eating the food is broken down into glucose. Generally foods that are high in fiber tend to be low on the glycemic index, as fiber slows the breakdown of sugars into the bloodstream. Because most vegetables are high in fiber, low on the glycemic index, and are packed with nutritional value, vegetables are an ideal way to meet your daily carbohydrate requirements.

Vegetables contain the majority of the micronutrients (vitamins, minerals, fiber and phytochemicals) your body needs. However, there are essential macronutrients vegetables cannot provide sufficient quantities of, including protein with all eight essential amino acids found only in animal products, and certain fats such as omega-3 with EHA and DPA fatty acids. Vegetables also contain a host of essential nutrients that are not found or replicated in any other type of food, and certainly not in any pill or supplement. They contain phytochemicals, for instance, which are used by the body to repair and build healthy cells, organs and tissues, thereby increasing your immunity to disease and illness. They are also rich in fiber, which aids in digestion and also creates a feeling of being full. Advocates of high grain-consumption, such as the USDA, often cite grain's fiber content when pushing the "need for grains," ignoring all its harmful effects. Vegetables are a far healthier choice than grains to obtain your fiber.

In short, vegetables provide tremendous health benefits. Vegetables' health benefits include, but are by no means limited to:

- Helping you to prevent disease
- Aiding you in healing existing disease
- Optimizing your weight
- Preventing wrinkles and restoring your youthfulness
- Increasing your energy, mental clarity and focus by leaps and bounds
- Improving your emotional health, including helping to fight depression
- Helping you live longer

What's more, vegetables can really taste incredible. My patients frequently tell me that soon after they stopped eating junk food, they stopped craving sugar and looked forward to eating vegetables and healthy protein. If you commit yourself to the dietary program according to your metabolic type as described in the "Pulling it All Together" section of this book, it's likely you'll have the same experience as many of my patients—that sugar tastes "sickeningly" sweet and that you've grown to love the taste of nature's bounty.

There are some important guidelines to consider in your vegetable selection, as not all vegetables are created equal:

1) Vegetables rich in color generally indicate that they are higher in vital nutrients than their pale counterparts. For example, dark green romaine lettuce, spinach or kale is much higher in nutrients than nearly white iceberg lettuce, which has virtually no nutritional value. Red onions are much higher in flavonoids and antioxidants than white or yellow onions. The same is true for red grapes versus green grapes, and red, yellow and purple bell peppers are higher in nutrients than green peppers and well worth the additional cost. There are some exceptions to this rule such as cauliflower, which is white but which is still a nutrient-dense vegetable.

2) For purposes of your health, pretend that potatoes are not a vegetable but a grain. That is because they are high in simple carbs and they act upon your body similar to grains and sugars, promoting weight gain and disease. This is true whether they are baked, mashed, boiled, or fried. Fried potatoes such as French fries are double trouble and you should avoid them like the plague. French fries are high in dangerous trans-fats, which are fats damaged by the heating process that contain a molecular conformation that causes heart disease and cancer. In addition, fried potatoes contain the carcinogenic substance acrylamide. Moreover, a Super Size French fry at McDonalds is 540 calories, 68 grams of carbohydrate, and 26 grams of fat—enough carbs and fat for an entire day! You would have to run at a fast pace for over an hour straight just to break even. In summary, I would not feed French fries to a starving dog much less a human.

3) Limit your consumption of other root vegetables, such as beets and carrots, as they are higher in carbohydrates than above-ground vegetables. If you do eat them, eat them raw as cooking increases their glycemic index.

4) Organic produce is usually much higher in nutrients and you'll also find organic produce tastes better. Plus, organic farmers don't use chemical fertilizers, pesticides or herbicides, all of which can harm your health. If you can't buy organic produce, don't let that stop you from buying produce at all, of course—just make sure you remove some of the chemicals by soaking them for 10 minutes in a sink with water, vinegar and hydrogen peroxide, or in a vegetable wash found at most health food stores.

5) Focus on eating your vegetables raw. Some people find raw vegetables difficult to digest and will have to incorporate them slowly and in small amounts. The reason for eating raw veggies is there are valuable and highly perishable micronutrients that are damaged when you heat them. Recipes for raw foods, vegetable juicing, salads and cooked vegetable dishes have been provided in this book to make eating vegetables easy for you.

Juicing Your Veggies

Juicing continues to grow in popularity in the U.S. because it is a convenient and delicious way to consume raw vegetables. This book provides you tasty and nutritious juicing combinations, but you should also experiment to find out which vegetables you prefer with other vegetables.

When it comes to juicing, though, the one tool that matters most is your equipment. If you are new to juicing you should first consider purchasing an inexpensive juicer or even a used juicer at a garage sale or on eBay. This will allow you to confirm that juicing is something you want to continue with. When you are certain you want to commit to juicing for the long-term, though, you'll want a higher quality machine. I compiled an extensive juicer comparison table evaluating the major brands and types of juicers. To see this table, go to Mercola.com and type in "juicing" in the search engine. Hands-down, the best juicer on the market in terms of value, durability, performance, and ease-of-use is the Omega 8002 Juicer. Beyond juicing, it is also designed for mincing, chopping, and more, and while comparable juicers cost $800–$2,000, the Omega 8002 Juicer is a tremendous value at $260. I personally have used the Omega 8002 Juicer since 2000 and I love it.

Limit the Legumes

Legumes such as lentils and navy, pinto, kidney, and black-eyed peas have significantly high levels of carbohydrates that can increase insulin levels. Therefore, those who are overweight, have high blood pressure, high cholesterol levels, or diabetes should avoid or significantly restrict their legume intake.

If you do not have insulin challenges, then legumes, in moderation, can be a nutritious food source as they are rich in both fiber and minerals. Legumes are also high in vegetable protein, but you should be aware that their protein is incomplete, as it does not contain all eight of the essential amino acids your body needs. Animal protein such as fish, meat, eggs, and dairy is the only source of complete protein and therefore vegetarians should consume some animal protein like dairy, non-toxic fish, or eggs to prevent protein deficiency. It is especially important for Protein Metabolic Types to consume adequate protein, as I have seen in my clinical practice Protein Types who developed serious illnesses from their vegetarian diets.

Soy Untrue!

Soybeans are another legume, but deserve their own special mention because of the extreme misperceptions of their supposed health value. There are a large number of companies seeking to profit from the alleged health benefits of soy, such as soy milk, powders, cheese, breakfast bars, cereals and nuts. The truth of the matter is that these products largely do more harm than good. "But what about the link between soy and the low rates of breast, colon and prostate cancer among Asian people, whose diets tend to be high in soy?" you may ask. Consider that Asians eat a diet that includes significantly higher quantities of vegetables and much lower quantities of processed foods, and a much better balance of omega-3 to omega-6 fat ratios. Asians as a whole are consuming a far healthier diet overall, which provides relative protection from the harmful effects of soy. It should also be noted that Asians eat a significant portion of soy in the recommended fermented form such as natto, amakaze, miso and tempeh, which nullifies the negative effects of soy. While an entire recently published and excellent book is available on how soy can harm yur health, *The Whole Soy Story* by Dr. Kaayla Daniel, here are some essentials you should know:

- Soybeans are high in natural toxins, also known as "antinutrients." This includes a large quantity of inhibitors that deter the enzymes needed for protein digestion. Further, these enzyme inhibitors are not entirely disabled during ordinary cooking. The result is extensive gastric distress and chronic deficiencies in amino acid uptake, which can result in pancreatic impairment and cancer.

- Soybeans contain hemaglutinin, which causes red blood cells to clump together. Soybeans also have growth depressant substances. And while these substances are reduced in processing, they are not completely eliminated.

- Soy contains goitrogens, which frequently lead to depressed thyroid function.

- Most soybeans are genetically modified, and they contain one of the highest levels of pesticide contamination of all foods.

- Soybeans are very high in phytates, which prevent the absorption of minerals including calcium, magnesium, iron and zinc, all of which are co-factors for optimal biochemistry in the body. Eating meat reduces the mineral-blocking effects of these phytates, and so it is helpful if you do eat soy to also eat meat.

- Finally, in an effort to remove the antinutrients from soy, soybeans are taken through a series of chemical processes including acid washing in aluminum tanks. This leaches high levels of aluminum, a toxic heavy metal, into the final soy products. Many soy foods also have toxic levels of manganese. Soy formula has up to 80 times higher manganese than is found in human breast milk.

There are additional concerns about soy if you are pregnant or intend to be, as nearly 20% of all infants are now fed soy formula. Visit the very popular and always-expanding article entitled "Why Soy Can Damage Your Health" on Mercola.com, which will link you to over twenty-five different articles and their corresponding studies on the risks of soy, which far outweigh any benefits.

Be Only Moderately Fruit-ful

Fruits, while high in vitamins and antioxidants, are also higher in sugar content than vegetables. If you are trying to lose weight, or have high blood pressure or diabetes, it is wise to omit fruits from your diet or restrict yourself to eating a small handful of berries a day. This is especially true if you are a Protein Type with the above conditions as most fruit is not beneficial for Protein Types. One exception of this is coconut, which provides the high fat content Protein Types need. Carb Types tend to do much better with fruits, especially citrus fruits such as oranges and grapefruits, and can consume a moderate amount.

In selecting fruit, berries such as blueberries, raspberries, lingonberries, bilberries, cranberries and black currants should be amongst your top choices because they have, relative to other fruits, a lower quantity of sugar while providing high vitamin C, dietary fiber, folic acid, and phytochemicals. They provide excellent protection against heart disease and cancer. They also can help prevent and treat vision problems.

Amongst the best of all berries are blueberries. They are quite low in sugar compared to other fruits yet pack some of the most powerful antioxidant properties of all fruits and vegetables. In addition to preventing heart disease, cancer, and other diseases, they've been shown to slow the aging process, especially in the brain. (For an exceptional source of organic blueberries that taste incredible and that you can get delivered to you year-round, check out the "Recommended Ingredients and Products Locator" in the Appendix.)

On a final note, be especially careful about consuming hybrid fruits. Hybrids are foods altered by humans to "improve" upon them, and they therefore can't grow in nature. In the case of fruits, "improve" usually has meant, among other factors, increasing their sugar content so they taste even sweeter. Fruits that don't contain seeds (but naturally should) are, for example, hybrids. That means you should steer clear of seedless oranges, seedless watermelon, seedless grapes, and other produce labels that boast of being "seedless." It almost always indicates they have even higher sugar content, which can impair your health.

The High-Standing Coconut

Coconut, the "fruit" of the palm tree, is an exceptionally nutritious food that offers many benefits including helping you fight and prevent disease, and helping you lose weight and keep it off. Coconut meat is a particularly smart choice for Protein Types, as it is high in protein. Islanders have long been prized coconuts for their preventive and curative powers over disease and illness, and this is primarily because they are rich in lauric acid, a proven antiviral, antibacterial and antifungal agent.

Coconuts are high in saturated fat that, contrary to popular belief, is a necessary fat for optimal nutrition. There are three different types of saturated fats, and coconuts contain the healthiest type with medium-chain fatty acids that *will actually help you lose weight while increasing health!*

The medium-chain fatty acids (MCFA) abundant in coconuts are digested more easily and utilized differently by the body than other fats. Whereas other fats are stored in the body's cells, the MCFA in coconut oil is sent directly to the liver where it is immediately converted into energy. So when you eat coconuts and coconut oil your body uses it immediately to make energy rather than store it as body fat. Because this quick and easy absorption puts less strain on the pancreas, liver and digestive system, the oil in coconuts "heat up" your metabolic system. Since the coconut oil actually speeds up metabolism, your body will burn more calories in a day—this will contribute to weight loss, and you'll have more energy. Meanwhile, studies have shown the opposite for excessive omega-6 unsaturated fats such as canola, safflower, sunflower, corn, and vegetable oils: they can contribute to hypothyroidism and lower your metabolic rate.

Coconuts are high in protein and low in carbs. They are also good sources of folic acid, all B vitamins, and minerals including calcium, magnesium, and potassium.

Be Sane with Nuts

Eating moderate amounts of nuts has been shown to reduce the risk of type 2 diabetes, heart disease and cancer. What is more, nuts are a good source of protein. With their high protein and fat content, they are helpful at curbing hunger, which is why they are the cuisine of choice on airlines. But go easy on the nuts, as—except for walnuts—they are high in omega-6 fats that can unbalance your omega-6 to omega-3 ratio, which can have profound negative health consequences (you can visit my site for more information on this vitally important topic.) The high fat content of nuts is also, in my experience, an easy fuel for weight gain, so those with weight issues may want to avoid them.

Walnuts, similar to flaxseeds, are relatively high in omega-3, an essential nutrient that most Americans are sorely lacking in their diet but that has a profound impact on keeping cholesterol levels in check, preventing heart disease and cancer, aiding in depression, and more. The best type of omega-3 fats, EPA (Eicosapentaenoic Acid) and DHA (Docosahexaenoic Acid), are found in the oils in fish and are crucial to optimal health. DHA and EPA, for instance, are pivotal to preventing depression, schizophrenia, memory loss, and Alzheimer's disease. On the other hand, the omega-3 in walnuts contains alpha-linolenic acid (ALA), an omega-3 fat that helps prevent abnormal heart rhythms and has been shown to cut the risk of sudden cardiac death among people who have already suffered a heart attack. Furthermore, walnuts contain ellagic acid, an antimutagen, anticarcinogen, and cancer inhibitor.

Other types of nuts like almonds and pecans, while high in omega-6, can still be good if used in moderation, as they also have heart disease- and cancer-preventing properties. Protein Types in particular can benefit from eating a few small handfuls a week, either within recipes or as a snack. Again, though, if you are trying to lose weight, rigidly restrict your consumption of fattening nuts—at most, sprinkle them on salads or in recipes for enhancement.

As for the ever-popular peanut (actually a legume, but nutritionally much closer to nuts), it is associated with reducing the risk of heart disease and is high in protein. But you must use be careful not to consume excessive amounts of peanuts, as they are loaded with omega-6 fats. Moreover, peanut crops can be contaminated with a carcinogenic mold toxin called aflatoxin, and they have the highest pesticide residues of any crop. If you want the health benefits of peanuts without the high level of risk, look for the "Arrowhead Mills" brand of organic peanut butter in stores. The peanuts they use are grown in New Mexico, where aflatoxin has not been reported as a problem due to the dry conditions, and their organic peanut butter is free of pesticides. Additionally, when you open the jar, you can pour off the oil that has settled on top of the peanut butter rather than stirring it in, which will lower the omega-6 content and further improve the vitally important omega-3:6 ratio.

Selective Seeds

As with nuts, seeds can offer myriad health benefits, but if you are overweight you should limit your seed consumption as they can contribute to weight gain.

One prominent exception to the weight issue is flaxseed, which has been shown to promote weight loss, decrease cholesterol levels, and aid in digestion. Flaxseed can also lower the risk of heart attack and stroke by helping to keep the arteries free of plaque and cholesterol.

Flaxseeds, which can be found in most health food stores, are exceptionally high in omega-3 with ALA, which enhances your immune system and protects against a variety of diseases. Please remember, however, that you still need the omega-3 with DHA and EPA, found only in fish oils. Flaxseeds can be ground in a coffee grinder or other types of grinders and used in a variety of recipes. Be cautious, though, about consuming flaxseed oil, as it is relatively unstable oil that most people don't seem to tolerate well.

Sesame, pumpkin and squash seeds are fair choices for snacking, but should be used in limited amounts as they are relatively high in omega-6 fats and will alter the omega-3:6 ratio. Additionally, those with weight issues should consume only very low amounts at best. Sesame seeds are high in protein, B vitamins, calcium, copper, iron, magnesium, phosphorous and zinc. Sesame seeds, containing a variety of amino acids, are especially good for heart health and improving endurance. Tahini, a popular spread made from sesame seeds and used in several recipes in this book, can be found in most health food stores.

Pumpkin and squash seeds are high in iron, phosphorous, fiber, and protein. They also contain high amounts of zinc that may offer some protection against the development of prostate cancer. You are far better off choosing the raw variety of pumpkin and squash seeds, as roasting seeds damages their delicate essential fatty acids. Fats that are damaged end up as the building blocks for hardening of your arteries.

The Slickest Oils

Besides grains and sugars, there is no category of food that the public has received more dangerous half-truths about than edible oils. An imperative piece of advice for you to follow is to limit the omega-6 fats and trans-fats in your diet. Trans-fats are primarily formed when vegetable oils are "hydrogenated" or "partially hydrogenated," which means that the oil was heated as such high temperatures that it changed the structure of the molecule so that it is more stable at room temperature (at the expense of being harmful to the body.) So look for those words when you read ingredient labels and avoid those products. Unfortunately, trans-fats are found in most packaged processed foods, such as baked goods, cereals, cookies, crackers, soup mixes, frozen foods and fried foods like French fries, tortilla chips and doughnuts. Trans-fats lead to clogged arteries, heart disease, and because they lower the "good" cholesterol, they indirectly lead to high cholesterol.

Fortunately, the danger of trans-fats is starting to receive widespread publicity, and in the near future it seems likely trans-fats will be widely recognized as a leading food toxin to shun in the mainstream mind. It's not soon enough, but the FDA has mandated that trans-fat content must be listed on all nutrition labels by 2006.

A major health hazard of corn, safflower and the other unsaturated oils once pushed as "heart healthy" is that they are very high in omega-6 fatty acids. For quite some time, the American public was convinced that unsaturated oils were the darlings of a healthy diet, while oils high in saturated fats were the enemy of health. The "evil" saturated fats include: coconut oil, butter, and red meat. The history of this drastically incorrect perception is fascinating, and points directly to how government and the food industry can, largely in the quest for profit and power, harm the public health. This history, as well as extensive insight on why saturated fats are actually essential to your health, is covered well in the book *Know Your Fats: The Complete Primer for Understanding the Nutrition of Fats, Oils and Cholesterol*, by Mary Enig, Ph.D., the nation's leading expert on fats and oils.

According to Enig, back in the early 1950s, and based only on very partial and inconclusive research, several government and other influential health organizations proposed that the conventional diet that included saturated fats from products like butter, meat and coconut oil was dangerous to the heart. Even at that time, though, many studies contradicted this assumption, and other nations whose diets had a saturated fat intake higher than Americans were not experiencing near the same rate of heart disease—but this information was largely ignored. The food manufacturers of margarine and corn, safflower, sunflower, and other monounsaturated oils took advantage of the misperception, equating saturated fat with pure evil while promoting their products as essential health foods. Wesson, for instance, promoted its cooking oil as good "for your heart's sake." And as often happens with the onslaught of corporate marketing plus an inefficient government pushed by the special interests, myth became reality and the general public embraced the unsaturated and hydrogenated fats while shunning detrimental saturated fats. Of course, this turn towards the omega-6 oils and hydrogenated fats has contributed to the skyrocketing cases of heart disease and cancer, the number one and two killers in the U.S. respectively, and the overweight epidemic.

Subsequently, I strongly encourage you to reduce or eliminate your intake of nearly all vegetable oils, including corn, safflower, sunflower, canola, sesame and soybean oil, and related products such as margarine and vegetable shortening. You most certainly want to avoid cooking with these oils, as they are damaged by heat and turn into trans-fat; the only oil that is not damaged by cooking at higher temperatures that I am aware of is coconut oil. In addition to the trans-fat issue, these vegetable oils may suppress your immune system; in fact, vegetable oils are emulsified with water and injected in patients who have had organ transplants specifically to suppress their immune system. They can also cause oxidative damage, interfere with normal thyroid function, and further disrupt most people's already skewed omega-6 to omega-3 ratios.

Instead, the two best oils are coconut oil and extra-virgin olive oil. Olive oil is a monounsaturated fat and contains major benefits because of its vitamin E and A, chlorophyll, magnesium, squalene and a host of other cardio-protective nutrients. Unlike other oils, olive oil possesses these health benefits because it is unrefined and unheated. Olive oil has also been shown to reduce the risk of some cancers and rheumatoid arthritis. Additionally, olive oil is an omega-9 fatty acid and therefore it does not overload the body with omega-6 fats. However, a drawback to olive oil is that it is more susceptible to oxidative damage than coconut oil when cooked since it is a monounsaturated fat. The best bet with olive oil is to use it on salads, and use coconut oil for your cooking.

Coconut oil is abundantly nutritious and useful. It is a saturated fat that is better for cooking because it is stable at high temperatures. Coconut oil can also help you prevent and fight many diseases and illnesses. And, despite being a saturated fat, it can actually contribute to weight loss. Please refer to "The High-Standing Coconut" section earlier in this chapter, as all the benefits of eating coconut apply to coconut oil, as well.

Coconut oil is particularly recommended for those with diabetes. It helps regulate blood sugar, thus lessening the effects of the disease, and it also raises metabolic rate causing the body to burn up more calories and thus promoting weight loss. Since 1980, researchers have also demonstrated the benefits of coconut oil with Crohn's Disease and IBS, acting as an anti-inflammatory in the digestive tract. Its antimicrobial properties also promote intestinal health by killing troublesome microorganisms that may cause chronic inflammation.

What is more, applying coconut oil topically is exceptional for keeping your skin young and healthy as it protects against destructive free-radical formation in the skin cells. I have even had patients rub it on the bottom of their feet to eliminate hard dry skin there. Coconut oil can help to keep the skin from developing liver spots and other blemishes caused by aging and over exposure to sunlight, and it also helps to prevent sagging and wrinkling by keeping connective tissues strong and supple. In some cases it restores damaged or diseased skin.

There is really only one catch with coconut oil—you have to be very careful of the brand and type you choose. From brand to brand there is a very wide variance in quality due to factors such as the types of coconuts used, the manufacturing process employed to make the oil, and more, which will have a major impact on its healthiness and effectiveness. Your coconut oil should meet all of these standards:

- Certified organic, USDA standards
- No refining
- No chemicals added
- No bleaching
- No deodorization
- No hydrogenation
- Non-GMO
- From traditional palms only—no hybrid varieties
- From fresh coconuts, not the dried "copra" used in most coconut oils
- Low-level heated only so it does not damage nutrients

If you can't find high-quality virgin coconut oils meeting these standards in your local health food stores, check out Mercola.com, as I have extensively researched this subject and I have found an excellent brand meeting all of the standards above that can be shipped directly to you. Finally, it is worth repeating that the excellent health benefits of coconut oil can also be achieved through eating fresh raw coconuts, as covered earlier.

Bent on Fermented Foods

Traditionally fermented foods—a category that can include both plant- and animal-based foods, which is why this section bridges this chapter and the next—are a must in any healthy diet. Food fermentation is an ancient preparation and preservation technique produced through the breakdown of carbohydrates and proteins by microorganisms such as bacteria, yeasts and molds, and it makes foods taste delicious. Even more importantly, fermented foods are beneficial to overall health because they are probiotics, meaning they promote the growth of friendly intestinal bacteria, therefore aiding digestion and supporting immune function. This includes an increase in B vitamins (even vitamin B12), omega-3 fatty acids, digestive enzymes, lactase and lactic acid, and other immune chemicals that fight off harmful bacteria and even cancer cells. Fermented foods are so important, in fact, that they are a standard part of my dietary prescription to my patients.

It is important, though, to understand and beware the big difference between healthy fermented foods versus the commercially processed "imposter" versions. Fermentation is an inconsistent process—almost more of an art than a science—so commercial food processors developed techniques to help standardize more consistent yields. Technically, anything that is allowed to sit at room temperature in a salt solution to allow healthy bacteria to culture is fermented, but that's where the similarity ends, as each type of fermented food has unique requirements and production methods. Refrigeration, high-heat pasteurization and vinegar's acidic pH all slow or halt the fermentation and enzymatic processes.

"If you leave a jar of pickles that is still fermenting at room temperature on the kitchen counter," explains Richard Henschel of Pickle Packers International, "they will continue to ferment and produce carbon-dioxide, possibly blowing off the lid or exploding the jar—" which is why, of course, all "shelf-stable" pickles are pasteurized.

It is probably not surprising that our culture has traded many of the benefits of these healthy foods for the convenience of mass-produced pickles and other cultured foods. Some olives, such as most canned California-style black olives, for instance, are not generally fermented, but are simply treated with lye to remove the bitterness, packed in salt and canned. Olive producers can now hold olives in salt-free brines by using an acidic solution of lactic acid, acetic acid, sodium benzoate and potassium sorbate, a long way off from the old time natural lactic-acid fermenting method of salt alone. Some pickles, meanwhile, are simply packed in salt, vinegar and pasteurized. Most yogurts are so laden with sugar that they are little more than puddings. Unfortunately, these modern techniques effectively kill off all the lactic acid-producing bacteria and short-circuit their important and traditional contribution to intestinal and overall health.

You can still find some healthy traditional varieties of "lacto-fermented" (meaning the lactic acid producing abilities are intact) foods, however. The stronger-flavored, traditional Greek olives you are most likely to find on olive bars are not lye-treated and are still alive with active cultures. Generally so are the barrel-fresh pickles made in local delis every few days. But to be sure you are getting the great health benefits of these active, fermentation cultures, you should commit to routinely making lacto-fermented foods on your own. Olives, sauerkraut, miso, and crème fraîche are just some of the fermented recipes and ingredients you can find and easily make in Part Two of this book.

If you are seeking a highly convenient way to get the full health value of lacto-fermented foods, you should also consider a top-quality fermented food "kit." While these are quite popular in other parts of the world where the exceptional nutritional value of traditional fermented foods are well understood, they are still difficult to find in North America. But I have found a premier-quality "Kefir Starter" kit and "Culture Starter" kit that you can read more about in the "Recommended Ingredients and Product Locator" in the Appendix and conveniently order through the "Recommended Products" section of Mercola.com. Kefir, as you will read more about in the Dairy section of the next chapter, is one of the healthiest and delicious forms of lacto-fermented foods when made properly. Its taste and texture can best be compared to a more drinkable form of yogurt, and the Kefir Starter product makes creating it almost ridiculously simple. The "Culture Starter" product, meanwhile, is a very easy way to make cultured vegetables and even sour cream (i.e., traditionally fermented foods, not the unhealthy "imposter" versions on almost all grocery store shelves). Finally, for more on the incredible health necessity of fermented foods/probiotics in your diet, be sure to subscribe to the "Body Ecology Diet" e-newsletter at bodyecologydiet.com (see Appendix).

4: Animal-Based Foods: Mercola's Guide to the Healthiest

Meat Worth the Eat

Everyone—all metabolic types—need *good* protein. Carb Types need some, Mixed Types need more, and Protein Types need considerably more, as you'll learn in Chapter 5. The best source of protein is meat. Does this mean vegetarians shouldn't be vegetarians? No, but if you are a vegetarian, be sure to get include protein from dairy, eggs and fish, as only animal proteins provide all the essential amino acids and micronutrients your body requires to function at its highest level.

In order to fight and avoid disease, increase energy, and live longer, choosing the right *type* of meat is critical. It is all too easy to opt for the extreme convenience of heading to your local grocery store for their super-value-priced beef, chicken, or turkey, but this convenience is one of the most severe health mistakes you can make; it is much like building a house from sticks—sure they are cheap and easy to find, but you'll pay for it many, many times over in the end. **Perhaps more than any other type of food group, it is crucial to investigate how the meat you eat was raised.**

Let's start with the most popular meat, the beef you'll find in most grocery stores and served in almost all restaurants. The cattle slaughtered for this beef are, hands down, the unhealthiest creatures on earth. Their natural, biological diet is grass, but in order to raise more of them in a confined space, fatten them up to levels far higher than is natural, and get them to market much quicker, they are fed an unnatural diet of corn and other grains. Cows have a difficult time digesting grains as their physiology is designed for grass, and many would get sick and quickly die due to an overgrowth of deadly bacteria in their stomach that results from the grain they were never designed to eat. The factory farms therefore administer substantial amounts of antibiotics to prevent this. Long-term, high-dose antibiotic use in cattle (and in people who eat the antibiotic-laden meat) contributes to the formation of antibiotic-resistant bacteria, or "superbugs," which is a frightening problem indeed. There is still more: the giant agribusiness corporations like to get the cattle to market even quicker than this artificial grain diet enables, because it means even more profit, and so these cattle are also fed steroids. Furthermore, the grains they are fed are laced with pesticides and herbicides, and are genetically modified. What this all means is, with every juicy bite of a typical hamburger or steak, you are also eating an artificial concoction of vaccines, steroids, pesticides, herbicides, and GMO grains. Even worse, cattle's unhealthy grain diet, high in omega-6, strips beef of much of its nutritional value, including depleting the omega-3 fatty acids and conjugated linolenic acid (CLA) that you require to fight cancer and many other diseases.

Fortunately, there are a variety of healthy and delicious red meats available, such as bison and grass-fed beef, but before delving into those, let's address a couple of myths.

As mentioned previously, the saturated fat associated with red meat is not "evil." As top researchers, including Linus Pauling, Russell Smith, George Mann, John Yudkin, Abram Hoffer and Mary Enig have pointed out, your body actually requires moderate levels of saturated fat to protect the arteries, process calcium, stimulate the immune system, and add structural stability to the cell and intestinal walls. Dr. Enig, author of *Know Your Fats: The Complete Primer for Understanding the Nutrition of Fats, Oils and Cholesterol*, cites study after study supporting the contention that saturated fats are not harmful but, instead, it is most vegetable oils that are.

One of the contributors to the misconception that red meat is unhealthy was a study published in 1970 that reported that *processed* red meat, such as cold cuts, and *charred* red meat was harmful to health. But then, any sort of processed meat or meat that is black and crusty is not healthy, especially when it is raised in an unhealthy manner described above. To put the myths of saturated fat and red meat to rest once and for all, consider this: populations that eat a diet rich in fresh, natural red meat show far lower levels of high cholesterol and cancer, among other diseases. For much more information, including sources of the research, just type in "saturated fats" on the search engine of Mercola.com.

In terms of the red meats you can eat with confidence, grass-fed bison takes first prize as an outstanding health value plus what most people agree is an incredible taste. Meanwhile, bison is high in protein while containing fewer calories than an equivalent amount of skinless chicken or turkey. Bison is increasing in popularity here in the U.S. for obvious reasons, and so you may also be able to find it in finer grocery stores or health food stores, or you can find a great source for bison on Mercola.com.

Ostrich is an increasingly popular red meat that runs a close second in terms of taste and nutritional value, as it is also high in protein but has fewer calories than chicken and turkey. Although the big bird is a red meat, it tastes just like chicken and you can use it in place of beef or dark chicken meat in any recipe.

(Note: In the Bible, in Leviticus 11, ostrich is mentioned as one on a long list of animals that should not be consumed. While it does not explain why, and suggested explanations from clergy vary widely, it may refer to the fact that the wild ostrich's diet was unknown. Blackwing ostrich—the brand of ostrich I recommend—are fed on a diet primarily of the very healthy alfalfa, and free-range farmed in conditions far cleaner and healthier than the chicken, turkey and other meat commonly found in grocery stores. From a clinical perspective, I can highly recommend their ostrich as a very healthy meat. However, I personally believe the Bible is God's inherent word, including the Old Testament, so I choose to avoid eating ostrich and instead choose the equally healthy and delicious bison, and wanted to make sure others who may be concerned by this were aware, too.)

Another great source of wholesome protein is grass-fed beef. Because it is raised on the cattle's proper diet of grass, it is leaner than grain-fed beef. While the flavor is different than the fatty grain-fed beef many are used to, many of my patients come to prefer the taste of this lean grass-fed beef. With beef labeled as "grass-fed," though, you have to be careful as the cattle may only be "finished" on a diet of grass but fed grains for a majority of their lives. Make sure the grass-fed beef you choose is labeled as 100% grass-fed, and antibiotic-free. As a final point, lamb meat, though higher in fat than the meats previously listed, is also a healthy red meat option. With lamb and all other meats, you should ideally choose a grass-fed variety free of antibiotics, steroids, and other chemicals. I personally buy my lamb from the discount chain Costco because it is raised in Australia on green pastures of grass.

Meanwhile, the conventional white meats like chicken are not much better than the typical red meats found in grocery stores. Most store-bought chickens are raised in conditions where they can barely move throughout their entire lives. These inhumane conditions are not only heartrending, but also very unhealthy as they result in diseased chickens that are then given large doses of antibiotics. The birds are also raised on growth hormones to get them to market faster, and injected with moisturizing agents to make them taste "juicy." Furthermore, the chickens' diet consists of grains that are genetically modified and high in pesticides and herbicides.

The best white meats are free-range and certified organic chicken and turkey that contain no antibiotics, hormones or other chemicals. Turkey of this type can still be exceedingly expensive as it is more difficult to find, but free-range organic chicken is becoming quite popular and more affordable.

Wild game, such as venison, elk, rabbit, pheasant and quail, is another class of healthy meat to consider. Obviously, because they are wild, they are raised on their natural diets and have no artificial anything added. One drawback, though, is that there have been several cases of Mad Cow Disease reported in several types of wild game animals, particularly elk, but statistically your chances are still minute in encountering this problem. The other drawback is that many Americans are not accustomed to the "wild" taste of wild game. If you love the taste of "typical" beef and chicken, your best bets are the grass-fed bison and free-ranged chicken described above, which you'll find taste even better.

Something Fishy Going On

Fifty years ago, fish was probably the healthiest meat you could eat, as it is an exceptional protein source with the omega 3 fats DHA and EPA. Sadly in the last 50 years, the oceans and lakes have become polluted with hundreds of millions of tons of mercury primarily from burning coal for electricity. The mercury then bio-accumulates in the fish and makes eating fish a game of Russian roulette. Therefore, my best advice in descending order is:

1) Avoid eating any fish unless you know it has been laboratory-tested and proven to be free from mercury and other toxins

2) If you do eat fish that you are not sure has been laboratory-tested and proven to be free of toxins, at least choose from among the following six safest fish:

- Wild Pacific Salmon
- Tilapia
- Croaker
- Sardines
- Haddock
- Summer Flounder

3)   Eat fish sustainably harvested from the wild (such as the toxin-free Vital Choice salmon I discuss below), not "farm-raised." Because it is economical to fish farmers, farm-raised fish are fed grains like corn—obviously not their natural diet, as you don't see many fish swimming through Iowa's cornfields. These grains do not form the beneficial fatty acids DHA and EPA that are such an important reason to eat clean fish. Furthermore, farm-raised fish may also be exposed to tremendously high pesticide levels resulting from the run-off of nearby agricultural crops that are often heavily sprayed.

For the past 15 years, nutrition experts including myself, scientists, health organizations and the FDA have issued particular warnings against consumption of the larger fish like tuna, bass, halibut, swordfish, and marlin, which are higher on the food chain and therefore show the highest concentrations of mercury. In addition, many health experts, myself included, are now warning against any type of fish, as nearly all have toxic levels of mercury. In my own clinic, for example, we find many patients have high levels of mercury in their system, and we advise them to stop eating all fish except for those proven via laboratory testing to be safe. When they follow this advice I see a considerable reduction of their mercury levels on their laboratory analysis. There are other major causes of mercury toxicity, such as silver dental fillings and vaccines, but the primary cause is now fish.

It is very likely that an enormous number of Americans—and those from any country where fish is a routine meal—have dangerous levels of mercury in their system. The problem is, it's tasteless in fish, and does not "show itself" until it wreaks outright havoc on people's health. Mercury is easily absorbed and stubbornly retained by the body, and can result in damage to your brain and kidneys. Trace amounts of mercury in the system have been linked to Alzheimer's, Parkinson's, autism and several other neurological disorders. Fish consumption is particularly hazardous to pregnant women and children as the mercury can cause birth defects and harm the sensitive physiology of children.

Time for the good news! There are still some sources of fish that are safe from mercury and other toxins. Through independent laboratory testing, my team and I discovered one such source of wild Alaskan salmon, which you can find out more about and order through Mercola.com. Increasingly, I suspect health food stores will also be searching for and offering fish proven to be safe from mercury and other toxins, so you can also check with them. Again, your best bet is to ensure the fish has been lab-tested and shown safe, and your second best option is to at least stick to one of the six fish on the list above. Finally, though it's not a delicious meal option like mercury-free salmon, a convenient way to obtain the omega-3 with DHA and EPA fatty acids that your body needs is with a safe, purified fish oil, which I discuss thoroughly in Chapter 7.

The Great Egg Surprise

Eggs are one of the most nutritious foods on the planet, especially when consumed in their raw state. Some of you are now either recalling images of Sylvester Stallone in Rocky, or simply grimacing at the thought. But read on to understand why raw eggs are so healthy, and much safer than you might think.

Eggs, while being one of the best sources of good protein and fat, are also one of the foods that many people are allergic to. However, uncooked eggs have significantly lower allergic responses. This is because heating the egg protein actually changes its structural composition, and this distortion can easily lead to an egg allergy.

The typical concern about eating raw eggs is a fear of salmonella. But the risk of contracting salmonella from raw eggs is actually incredibly low. A recent study by the U.S. Department of Agriculture showed that of the 69 billion eggs produced annually, only 2.3 million of them are contaminated with salmonella. The translation is that only one in every 30,000 eggs is contaminated, which means that you are more likely to die in an airplane crash than contracting salmonella from raw eggs. Nevertheless, here are some suggestions on how to purchase the healthiest eggs possible.

Foremost, remember that healthy eggs come from healthy chickens, and unhealthy eggs from unhealthy chickens. Whether you eat your eggs raw or cooked, try to buy free-range organically fed, omega-3 enhanced eggs, which may be available in supermarkets, health food stores, or from local chicken farmers. Keep in mind that it is the conditions of commercial hens that are fed unclean diets and raised in small cramped cages where disease can easily spread. This makes the average supermarket eggs more likely to be infected with salmonella than eggs produced under healthy conditions. The following are additional steps to select healthy eggs:

3 Steps To Ensure Your Eggs Are Safe

1)   If you are getting your eggs fresh and un-refrigerated it is best to keep them on the counter at room temperature. (This will not work however if the eggs have already been refrigerated.) It is interesting to note that people do not refrigerate eggs in most other countries. One of the main reasons for keeping eggs at room temperature is that refrigeration causes slight damage to the egg protein.

2)   If there is a crack in the shell, don't eat it. You can easily check for this by immersing the egg in a pan of cool, salted water. If the egg emits a tiny stream of bubbles, don't consume it, as the shell is porous.

3)   Crack the egg open. A healthy egg has no foul odor, the egg white is gel-like (not watery), and a healthy egg yolk is convex and firm (not runny or bursts easily). If the egg does not have these characteristics, throw it away.

It is important to note that in the rare event that you do contract salmonella poisoning, you may feel sick and have loose stools, but this infection is easily treated by using high-quality probiotics that have plenty of good bacteria (discussed in detail in Chapter 7). You can take a one tablespoon of probiotics every 30 minutes until you start to feel better, and most people improve within a few hours.

Another concern is that raw egg whites contain a glycoprotein called avidin that is very effective at blocking biotin, one of the B vitamins, leading to a possible biotin deficiency. The solution to this is to consume eggs in their whole form (both egg yolks and whites) as the egg yolks contain high amounts of biotin to counteract avidin.

I've discovered a number of ways to make eating raw eggs enjoyable. You can mix them into any vegetable juice recipes you create. When you whip them up like a meringue, most people do not object to the texture, especially if there is a flavor added. You'll also find that by mixing flavorings like butterscotch or vanilla extracts with the eggs, and then adding raw milk or cream, you can create a delicious eggnog, and then you'll actually *enjoy and eagerly anticipate* the treat. Really! I have this eggnog for breakfast every day and I love it.

The Dairy Truth

The milk that is sold in grocery stores is *not* good for you, despite the onslaught of the National Dairy Council's "Got Milk?" marketing campaign with all their cute celebrity milk mustaches. That's because milk is literally processed to death by with pasteurization, which heats it at such high temperatures that it destroys microorganisms, good bacteria, live enzymes, vitamins and the delicate three-dimensional structure of the milk proteins. Conventional milk is also a problem because it comes from cows fed the unnatural diets of grain and is frequently injected with antibiotics and growth hormones to increase their milk production.

Pasteurization is a case of throwing out many babies with the bath water. This method of heating milk was first employed in the 1920s to kill germs leading to tuberculosis and other diseases linked to unclean production methods prevalent at the time. Unfortunately, milk pasteurization has many negative side effects:

- Kills beneficial enzymes including phosphatase, which allows the body to absorb calcium from the milk
- Destroys colloidal minerals, which are essential to absorb nutrients the milk would otherwise provide
- Precipitates minerals that cannot be absorbed by the body, contributing to osteoporosis
- Precipitates sugars that cannot be digested and fats that are toxic
- Destroys beneficial bacteria and lactic acids that help to protect your body against disease
- Diminishes the cortisone-like factor in the milk that would otherwise help combat allergies
- Destroys vitamins B12 and B6 in the milk
- Promotes other pathogens in the milk
- Contributes to allergies, osteoporosis, arthritis, heart disease, cancer, tooth decay, colic, disorders of the female reproductive system, and weakened immune systems

Milk pasteurization is a product of a bygone era, when controls were not in place for ensuring clean conditions for the cows, but the improved sanitation practices of the modern dairy industry have made pasteurization unnecessary.

The alternative is raw, organic, grass-fed milk. This is milk straight from the udders of grass-fed cows raised on their natural diets with no hormones. Raw milk is rich in glycol-sphingolipids (fats that aid in digestion) and conjugated linolenic acid (CLA), another type of fat that protects against cancer. Because it comes from grass-fed cows, it is rich in omega-3, and far richer than store-bought milk in the vitamins like A and D. Additionally, if infants are weaned from breast milk to raw cow (or goat's) milk, and they avoid fruit juice, most grains and sugars, there is a strong likelihood that they will avoid dental cavities.

Raw milk is, however, still illegal in many U.S. states. Why? Because pasteurization became mandatory law when cows were raised in unclean conditions. More so, it's because the National Dairy Council has a very powerful lobbying arm in Washington, D.C. and, because the powerful corporations they represent are entirely built around pasteurization, and they don't want raw milk to become legal again—if the truth gets out too far, after all, so goes their profits.

Fortunately, organizations like the Weston A. Price Foundation with their "Campaign for Real Milk" have been helping to promote the legalization of raw milk. As of this writing raw milk sales through cowshare programs are allowed in Alaska, Arizona, California, Illinois, Kansas, Maine, Massachusetts, Minnesota, Nebraska, Nevada, New Hampshire, New York, Oklahoma, Oregon, Pennsylvania, South Carolina, South Dakota, Texas, Utah, Vermont, Washington, and Wisconsin. All other states currently prohibit the sale of raw milk. The catch is, with the noteworthy exception of California, where it can be sold legally in stores, in most of these states you have to either find a small farmer who sells it, join a cowshare program, or—and this is only very recently—obtain your raw dairy from the one organization who has found a way to sell it legally throughout the U.S.

If you are interested in having raw milk, raw cream, and other dairy products shipped to you (and you live in the U.S.—other countries and regions within those countries have their own rules on the legality of raw dairy) from this organization, go to the "Recommended Products" section of www.Mercola.com and review the full listings for both the raw cheeses and the raw milk there. The cheeses under the raw cheese listing can be shipped rather inexpensively, but with the raw milk, cream and other dairy, keep in mind they are shipped frozen so unfortunately the shipping charges can be costly. Still, their dairy products are likely the healthiest (and most delicious) you will find anywhere, so it could be well worth the investment… especially if you are able to purchase it in bulk.

With cowshare programs, you become part owner of a cow and, on a routine basis, visit a specified location to pick up your share of raw milk. I'm a member of one such cowshare program in the Chicago area, and if you live in the Chicago area you can find out more by typing "raw milk" in the Mercola.com search engine. If you live in any other area, the best way to begin your search for raw milk and raw milk products is to visit the "Campaign for Real Milk" website at RealMilk.com. They list raw milk contacts in every state and also provide further exceptional insights on the issues and benefits of raw milk.

Other beneficial dairy products are unpasteurized butter, kefir, yogurt, and cheese from grass-fed cows. The beneficial bacterial found in yogurt and kefir is excellent for enhancing the digestive and immune system, but since yogurt and kefir found in most grocery stores has the same problems as pasteurized milk, it is best to make your own yogurt or kefir from raw milk.

Even though it is an ancient health food, many people today may not be familiar with kefir— but they should be. Traditionally lacto-fermented foods are an essential part of any diet as noted in the previous chapter (also see the recipes in "Raw, Sprouted and Fermented Foods" in Chapter 12), and kefir is among the most exceptional of such fermented foods. Meaning "feel good" in

Turkish, kefir is a cultured, enzyme-rich food filled with friendly microorganisms that will help balance your "inner ecosystem" and dramatically improve your immune system. Kefir's tart, refreshing flavor is similar to a drinking-style yogurt, but in addition to the gut-friendly probiotics found in yogurt, kefir contains highly beneficial yeast. When used regularly, the naturally occurring bacteria and yeast in kefir combine symbiotically to replenish the intestinal flora and provide you major protection against illness. Furthermore, those who have a dairy allergy or intolerance may be able to tolerate kefir as the fermentation process breaks down the lactose sugars in the milk and makes it much easier to digest.

Among its many restorative powers, kefir will:

- Provide supplemental nourishment for pregnant and nursing women
- Contribute to a healthy immune system and help fortify patients suffering from AIDS, chronic fatigue syndrome, herpes, and cancer
- Promote a tranquilizing effect on the nervous system and benefit many who suffer from sleep disorders, depression, and ADHD (attention deficit hyperactivity disorder)
- Help relieve all intestinal disorders, promote bowel movement, reduce flatulence, and create a healthier digestive system... **kefir is an absolute must after the use of antibiotics to restore balance to the digestive tract**
- Curb unhealthy food cravings by making the body more nourished and balanced

While you can find prepared kefir in some grocery stores, it bears repeating that you should use great caution with these brands. They are usually prepared with pasteurized milk and possibly other health-defeating processes and additional ingredients. Instead, I strongly urge you to use a "kefir kit" to quickly and easily make your own healthy kefir. I suspect such kits will be increasingly easy to find as word of this tremendous fermented health food spreads, but right now there is one kefir kit I highly recommend—the "Kefir Starter" by Body Ecology. You simply mix one packet of their starter to milk (again I recommend raw milk) or the juice of a young coconut and it's ready to go! You can find out more about this Kefir Starter and order through the "Recommended Products" section of Mercola.com, or ask your local health food store if they carry it.

And so finally, what about the dairy product so beloved in Western culture—cheese? Well, cheese made from conventional milk has all the problems with contamination that milk does, so if you eat cheese it is important to at least eat organic grass-fed cheese. Best of all, though, is raw milk cheese from organic grass-fed cows. The good news is that raw milk cheese is regulated differently than raw milk and is therefore relatively easier to find in health food stores. I strongly encourage you to check out the "Recommended Products" section of Mercola.com, though, as after much searching I have found an exceptional farm source for raw milk and organic grass-fed cheeses that will ship directly to you. They offer a wide choice of cheeses (cheddar, mozzarella, feta, brick and many more), and not only are they healthy, but they taste absolutely incredible!

5: The Dietary Key: Eat According to Your Metabolic Type

There is no one diet that is right for everyone. But there is a diet that is perfect for you. That means there is an ideal balance of food macronutrients—proteins, carbohydrates, fats—which you should consume for your specific biochemistry, as you'll learn in this chapter.

Once you discover your metabolic type and follow its corresponding dietary principles, you will experience noticeable improvements with your body and mind, just as my patients experience. If you are overweight, you will lose weight while feeling satisfied with eating, and you'll actually want to continue with the program (versus having to force yourself to, as with other diets). If you are an athlete, you will experience a major increase in all aspects of your game, including stamina, strength, balance, and concentration, and this increase will continue as you stick with the program. If you have a chronic disease, you will likely be addressing some of the underlying nutritional causes of your disorder, and so you will also notice an improvement in your symptoms.

While most of the diets that are currently popular are not centered carefully on maximizing health and prolonging life as my plan is, some do indeed at least effectively reduce weight—for some people. That is, if the diet is appropriate for their metabolic types. Have you ever wondered why two people can go on the same weight-loss diet and one loses weight (at least temporarily) while the other remains the same or gains weight? It is because people have different nutritional needs based on their individual biochemistry. If you are a Protein Type, for example, nutrients act very differently in your body than they do in a Carb Type. As the saying goes, one man's food can be another man's poison.

While medical practitioners and patients alike have been calling metabolic typing "revolutionary" and "the missing piece" in achieving optimal individualized nutrition, it is really just based on pure commonsense, as you'll learn below.

You're an Individual, You Need an Individualized Diet

Look around. You are unique. It's indisputable. Nobody looks exactly like you, and nobody ever has. Nobody speaks exactly like you, has the same gestures you do, or shares your fingerprints. No one thinks or feels exactly like you, either. So why do all the diets out there treat us like what's inside each of us is identical to what's inside everyone else? The one-size-fits-all approach to dieting is wrong because each of us is unique.

These metabolic differences are evident when we examine how people react differently to various amounts of protein, fat and carbs in their diets. Everyone has specific macronutritional needs that ranges from those who need a very high level of carbohydrates in their diet and a relatively low level of protein and fat (Carb Type), to those who need a very high level of protein and fat and a relatively low level of carbohydrates (Protein Type). After taking the test in this chapter, you will find that you fall into one of three general categories: Protein Type, Carb Type, or Mixed Type.

Your metabolic type is a general guide based on your answers from the metabolic typing questionnaire. Your metabolic type is not fixed or permanent and may change over time. It is important that you follow your MT recommendations as a starting place and pay attention to how your body feels, then make changes based on your experimentation and "listening to your body" to fine tune your food choices for optimal health.

The concept of using individual diets for individual people is certainly not new and has surfaced in many civilizations throughout time. For example, the ancient Greeks and Romans recognized that different people had different health requirements, thus leading to Lucretius' famous proclamation that "One man's food is another man's poison." Meanwhile, in the Far East, Chinese medicine taught that everyone has different constitutions (and therefore different dietary and treatment requirements) based on their unique characteristics and energetic imbalances. The 5,000-year-old Ayurvedic medicine of India identified three body types or doshas—pitta, vatta and kapha—each with their own specific dietary needs.

The concept for individualized diets has persisted since then, but in 1956 Dr. Roger Williams, a biochemist from the University of Texas, made a major advance in this concept with his classic book *Biochemical Individuality*. In it he noted that individuality pervades every part of the body, from how the organs function to the composition of body fluids. According to Williams, individuality extends to the cells, including the speed and efficiency with which cells perform their special functions. Furthermore, Williams noted that unbalanced or inadequate nutrition at the cellular level is a major cause of human disease, and that individuals have genetically determined and highly individualized nutritional requirements. Williams was the primary inspiration for Dr. William Kelley, an orthodontist with degrees in biology, chemistry and biochemistry who refined Williams' ideas into the first form of metabolic typing in the 1960s and 1970s. Kelley next incorporated Francis Pottenger, M.D.'s work into metabolic typing. Back in the 1930s and 40s, Pottenger had conducted research demonstrating that the autonomic nervous system played a central role in determining what types of foods and nutrients different people need.

William Wolcott—author of *The Metabolic Typing Diet*, now considered to be the authoritative book on the subject—then joined Kelly and together they experienced great clinical success at actually using metabolic typing to help improve patients' health. In the early 1980s Wolcott further refined metabolic typing through the influence of George Watson, Ph.D., a clinical psychologist and author of the book *Nutrition and Your Mind*. Dr. Watson had developed his own nutritional system based on people's metabolic differences, but his metabolic approach was based on cellular oxidation—the rate at which your cells convert nutrients into energy. Dr. Watson had noticed that some people were "fast oxidizers" who burned foods and nutrients quickly, while others were "slow oxidizers" who burned foods and nutrients slowly. Dr. Watson discovered that by prescribing specific foods and nutrients to balance oxidative imbalances in patients, many of their clinical problems were resolved.

Wolcott further refined the system by incorporating a host of other metabolic factors, the most prominent among them the endocrine system. Based on his clinical findings from working with thousands of patients, Wolcott designed an extensive questionnaire for determining metabolic type. In fact, I use this questionnaire with all my patients who come to my clinic, The Optimal Wellness Center. I have used metabolic typing with patients for the past two years. Before metabolic typing my program was teaching patients to eat natural, whole foods—the right forms of macronutrients—and to use techniques to improve their emotional well-being. Once I started to use metabolic typing, I recognized an amazing improvement in the rate of healing, health and vitality in my patients—and continue to witness it daily. Metabolic typing, I have come to realize, is essential to optimal health.

Metabolic typing is primarily based on the interrelationship between the body's autonomic nervous system and oxidative system. The autonomic nervous system controls all your involuntary muscles and functions, like heart rate, sweating, bowel movements, blinking and digestion, while the oxidative system is involved in converting nutrition to energy. Whatever control system is dominant in you determines your metabolic type.

If you are interested in a deeper analysis of the principles behind metabolic typing, I highly recommend William Wolcott's book, *The Metabolic Typing Diet*, available through the "Recommended Products" section of Mercola.com and on the shelves of many bookstores and libraries.

But the bottom-line is this: the answer to the right diet, right foods, and right nutrition for you ultimately resides within your genes, and metabolic typing provides the roadmap. If you want to optimize your weight, fight and prevent disease, increase energy and concentration, retain a youthful appearance, stop wasting tons of money on ineffective products and programs, and just feel better in general, a very effective and efficient way to do so is: 1) learn your metabolic type, 2) eat the healthy forms of foods and adopt the other healthy lifestyle approaches defined in this book, and 3) learn to "listen to your body" to eat the right balance of healthy foods for your metabolic type.

Determining Your Metabolic Type

The following test will give you a general idea of your metabolic type. It is important to point out that this is a very condensed version of the sophisticated and expansive clinical test that was designed by William Wolcott over a period of 30 years. Again, metabolic type exists on a spectrum; while the comprehensive clinical test is far more accurate and personalized, this abbreviated version still provides a reasonable point to start from. If you are interested in an even more reliable assessment of your type at a low cost, William Wolcott's previously mentioned book, The Metabolic Typing Diet, provides a more succinct 60-question test. Finally, if you are interested in taking the actual full professional test used in clinical offices, you can find out the convenient method of doing so in the note following the test below.

The most essential aspect of metabolic typing is to experiment with foods and pay attention to how they make you feel and to follow the diet that makes you feel your best. You'll learn all about these skills of "listening to your body" and "fine-tuning your diet" in the next section of this chapter, and the tips and notes in the recipes in this book have also been designed to help you toward this end.

General Test to Determine Your Basic Metabolic Type

For the following general test, simply answer the questions as honestly as you can, choosing the number that best represents your answer on the scale provided for each question. Remember, there are no right or wrong answers, and it's of course not "better" to be one type or another. If you don't know the answer to a question because you haven't tried a specific food yet, or don't remember how it affects you, then consume that food first and notice its effects on you, and then answer the question.

1) Does a high-carbohydrate meal or snack, one that is loaded with plenty of vegetables, bread, toast, cereals, rice, fruits, grains or potatoes, as the main food source satisfy your appetite, or stimulate it further?

1	2	3	4	5	6	7	8	9	10
satisfies									stimulates

2) When you eat a lot of red meat does it cause you to lose or gain body fat? Do you look slimmer in the mirror or is it easier for your clothes to fit?

1	2	3	4	5	6	7	8	9	10
gain weight									lose weight

3) Do you constantly think about food and frequently look forward with eager anticipation to your next meal or what you want to eat?

1	2	3	4	5	6	7	8	9	10
no									yes

4) What is your appetite like at breakfast, lunch and dinner?

breakfast...

1	2	3	4	5	6	7	8	9	10
weaker									stronger

lunch...

1	2	3	4	5	6	7	8	9	10
weaker									stronger

dinner...

1	2	3	4	5	6	7	8	9	10
weaker									stronger

5) Does eating something higher in fat and/or protein such as dark meats, avocados, cream, butter or coconuts within an hour or two of bedtime help you sleep better?

1	2	3	4	5	6	7	8	9	10
no									yes

6) If you ate a large salad with some low-fat meat like chicken breast for lunch (versus higher fat meat like a hamburger patty), how would it affect your productivity throughout the rest of the afternoon?

1	2	3	4	5	6	7	8	9	10
I'd have ample energy and feel satisfied								I'd become tired and hungy	

7) How often do you typically feel the need to eat on an average day? The extremes here would be feeling good with one meal scored as a 1, while needing 5 or 6 meals a day would place you at a 10. If you felt good on three meals a day that would be a 5.

1	2	3	4	5	6	7	8	9	10
1–2 times including snacks								5–6 times including snacks	

8) How much do you enjoy sour foods like pickles, sauerkraut, or vinegar?

1	2	3	4	5	6	7	8	9	10
love them									can't stand them

9) At Thanksgiving or a meal where you eat turkey, and assuming all the turkey is moist, if you prefer white meat give yourself a 1, if you only prefer the dark meat give yourself a 10, and if it doesn't matter give yourself a 5.

1	2	3	4	5	6	7	8	9	10
white meat									dark meat

Now add up each of the nine numbers you circled to get your total score, and your basic metabolic type:

- A score over 60 indicates a Protein Type. The higher your score above 60, the more likely you are truly a Protein Type.

- A score under 60 indicates a Carb Type. The lower your score under 60, the more likely you are truly a Carb Type.

- A score between 40 and 70 indicates a potential Mixed Type. If you scored in this range, you can begin fine-tuning your diet as explained below, but it is recommended that you take the more sophisticated test in William Wolcott's book, *The Metabolic Typing Diet*, to provide yourself a more reliable starting point.

[NOTE: The quiz above provides a very rough estimate of your metabolic type. Ultimately you will need to fine-tune whatever your results are anyway, but the advantage of the professional-level test used in clinical offices is that it can save you a considerable amount of time. If you are suffering from a serious health challenge like cancer or MS, you should seriously consider taking the more accurate clinical test in conjunction with an individualized consultation. This may save you up to six months of time in which your health may otherwise deteriorate significantly without professional assistance. You can go to **www.mercola.com/mttest.htm** to learn how to take the full clinical test easily and conveniently from your own home. The test consists of detailed questions that take about an hour to answer, and results in 1) a 24-page customized report on the foods and diet plan ideal for you and 2) a 45-minute one-on-one phone consultation with a trained Metabolic Type Advisor who will provide further insight on your personalized diet and answer questions you may have. At the time of this writing, though, this full clinical test and consequential personalized plan cost $179. I wanted to let you know this is the best option, and the next-best option is the 60-question test in Wolcott's book The Metabolic Typing Diet, which is more detailed than the test we have just provided.]

Listening to Your Body and Fine-Tuning Your Diet

You now have a general idea of your metabolic type. To understand the importance of listening to your body in order to fine-tune your ideal macronutrient level, imagine a line segmented into three parts: the first third of the line on the left is the Carb Type; the second third of the line in the middle is the Mixed Type; and the third part on the right is the Protein Type. You now know the basic area you reside in. However, you now want to figure out particularly where, today, you reside within your third of that line. For instance, are you a Protein Type who needs even more protein in your diet than the "average" Protein Type? Are you a Carb Type who needs somewhat less carbohydrates in your diet than the "average" Carb Type? This is where the simple but highly effective process of listening to your body and fine-tuning comes in.

First of all, there are specific proportions of carbs/fats/proteins recommended for each metabolic type. They are:

Carb Type: 25% Protein / 15% Fat / 60% Carbohydrate
Mixed Type: 30% Protein / 20% Fat / 50% Carbohydrate
Protein Type: 40% Protein / 30% Fat / 30% Carbohydrate

Use the percentages above as rough guidelines; occasionally you may want to calculate the percentage of protein, fat and carbs in your meals to see how your meals compare to the recommendations, but otherwise use the numbers above only in a general manner. If you are a Mixed Type, for instance, just think, "To start my diet, the food I eat on a daily basis should be around half good carbohydrates like vegetables and some fruits, with the other half as healthy proteins and fats like meat and dairy," (i.e., 50% carbs, 30% proteins, 20% fats.) And then do your best to aim for those general levels. The recipes in this book provide excellent guidelines to help you in this direction, but again, don't get compulsive about hitting the exact range—it is the process of listening to your body and fine-tuning, not following numbers on a page, that will be your primary guide in the process of honing in on your proper macronutrient level.

So what does "listening to your body" mean, first of all? Listening to your body means paying attention to how you feel, and for the purposes of fine-tuning your diet to determine your ideal macronutrient levels this means paying attention to how you feel up to two hours after you eat a meal. For instance, do you feel tired or mentally slow after a meal with your appropriate metabolic type ratios? If you feel sleepy 30–60 minutes after you eat, this is a giant clue that you ate the wrong types of food. This typically occurs when you eat too many carbs, especially grains. If your body is telling you it doesn't feel well after eating a meal you should experiment with varying the amount of carbs, fat, and protein and see how you feel. If after that meal your symptoms are even worse, then at the next meal (or at the same mealtime the next day) try varying the amount of carbs, fat, and protein in the other direction. This is the process of fine-tuning, and the goal is to find the proper ratio and proper forms of foods that allow to you feel your best, as defined in the following chart:

RIGHT MACRONUTRIENT RATIO	WRONG MACRONUTRIENT RATIO
you feel satisfied, not hungry or over-full	you may feel physically full but you're still hungry, or get hungry too soon again
you have no food cravings, especially sweets	you have food cravings such as for sweets or feel that something else was "missing" from the meal
you feel like your energy has been restored	you feel tired, lack energy, or too hyper, bouncing off the wall
your mind is clear and sharp	you can't focus well, you're spacey, or your mind is racing
you feel happy	you feel down, depressed, short-tempered, apathetic
any disease symptoms you have are either unchanged or improved	if you have a disease or disorder, your symptoms are sharper, worse

Reprinted with permission from The Metabolic Typing Diet: Customize Your Diet to Your Own Unique Body Chemistry *by William Wolcott, Doubleday Books, 2000*

Paying attention to your body's signals will require conscious effort and *self-trust* for the first several days, but you'll find it quickly becomes second nature. In fact, most people become so adept at this that they are able to rapidly discern the proportions, volume and type of macronutrients that are ideal for *them* at different points of the day (breakfast, lunch, dinner, snacks).

To help guide you in learning how to listen to your body after eating and fine-tune your diet accordingly, you can make copies of the "Fine-Tuning Your Diet to Your Metabolic Type Table" that has been included in the Appendix of this book. You can also print this table out from Mercola.com; simply enter "fine-tuning table" in the search engine there.

Food Guidelines for Each Metabolic Type

The following guidelines and recommended foods charts are based on over twenty years worth of clinical experience working with the metabolic types. These guidelines have proven true for most people, but again it is most important to pay attention to how the recommendations make you feel.

Carbohydrate Type

- For protein sources, emphasize low-fat, low-purine proteins such as chicken, ostrich, Cornish game hen and turkey breast. Only eat red meats occasionally.
- Monitor your reaction to dairy. Dairy is not ideal for you because Carb Types need to minimize calcium intake and dairy can throw your body out of balance. When eating dairy products you should strive for low-fat versions. If you consume raw milk, pour the cream off the top before consuming to reduce the fat content.
- Eat many vegetables, and focus on eating any vegetables that are not high in starch. High-starch vegetables to avoid include: potato, pumpkin, sweet potatoes, yams, corn, winter squash, carrots and beets. Include low-starch vegetables such as leafy greens, broccoli, tomatoes, peppers, and cabbage.
- Eat high-starch carbohydrates like legumes only in moderation.
- All fruits are fine; berries and citrus fruits are particularly good choices.
- You can eat whole grains in moderation, around 15% of your daily carb intake if you do not have overweight or obesity issues, diabetes, high cholesterol, or high blood pressure.
- While your proportion of protein is lower than other types, try to eat some protein with most meals to stabilize your blood sugar levels.
- Minimize your consumption of fats and oils. This does NOT mean a no-fat diet but simply that Carb Types do better on a low-fat diet.
- Eat the vegetable part of your meal first, as this will speed up your metabolic rate and oxidation, and then eat the protein and fat portion.

Carb Type Recommended Foods Table

Note: This table is not all-inclusive, but instead representative of the most highly recommended foods in relation with the other guidelines noted in the bullets above.

PROTEINS		CARBS		FATS / OILS	
meat	dairy	vegetables	fruit	nuts / seeds	fats / oils
low-fat, low-purine	non / low-fat	low-starch	all okay	use sparingly	use sparingly
chicken breast	grass-fed cheese	broccoli	apple	walnuts	butter
ostrich	raw milk	brussel sprouts	berries	flaxseeds	coconut oil
turkey breast	yogurt (raw milk)	cabbage	citrus fruit	pumpkin, squash	olive oil
cornish game hen	kefir (raw milk)	cucumber	grapes	sesame	
eggs		garlic	melons	sunflower	
lean pork		all leafy greens	peach, apricot	almonds	
		onions, scallions	pears	pecans	
		peppers	pineapple, tropicals	peanuts	
		sprouts	plums	coconuts	
		tomato		other nuts	
legumes	nuts / seeds	grains	legumes		
use sparingly	use sparingly	15% daily max whole grain only	use sparingly		

Protein Type

- Concentrate on high-density, high-purine proteins. These proteins are the dark meats of chicken and turkey and every protein that exists with the exception of: dairy, eggs, soy protein, and light meats like chicken and turkey breast, Cornish game hen, pork and lean ham.
- Salmon—as long as you know it has been laboratory tested and shown to be safe from mercury and other toxins—is also a good choice.
- Avoid grains and potatoes completely.
- Emphasize the following vegetables: asparagus, fresh green beans, cauliflower, spinach, celery, and mushrooms. These vegetables tweak your biochemistry in the proper direction.
- Limit the amount of fruits you consume because Protein Types tend to have blood sugar problems; coconuts, avocados, black and green olives, green apples, and pears are the best choices.
- Protein types tend to be hungrier than other types so be sure and snack as needed. Your snacks should include a protein food. Nuts like walnuts or dairy snacks like grass-fed cheese may work but if they leave you hungry or tired you will need to eat snacks with heavier protein like pate, lamb, or grass-fed beef.
- Protein Types are able to better support their fast metabolism by consuming a liberal amount of healthy fats and oils like butter, coconut oil, and olive oil, fats from animal based foods, and nuts.
- Alcohol in any form is especially bad for your type; you might feel a temporary lift after drinking it, but this will usually be followed by a major energy crash. Listen to your body and carefully moderate your alcohol intake or avoid it altogether.
- Eat the protein part of your meal first to slow down your oxidation rate, and then eat your vegetables.

Protein Type Recommended Foods Table

Note: This table is not all-inclusive, but instead representative of the most highly recommended foods in relation with the other guidelines noted in the bullets above.

PROTEINS		CARBS		FATS / OILS	
meat/fish	dairy	vegetables	fruit	nuts / seeds	fats / oils
high- and mid-purine	whole-fat	very low-starch	use moderately	all okay	all okay
livers, beef and chicken	grass-fed cheese	asparagus	avocados	walnuts	butter, cream
organ meats	raw milk	green beans, fresh	blueberries	coconuts	coconut oil
pates	raw cream	cauliflower	coconuts	flaxseeds	olive oil
grass-fed beef	yogurt (raw milk)	celery	olives	pumpkin, squash	
bison	kefir (raw milk)	mushrooms		sesame	
chicken, dark meat		spinach	use sparingly	sunflower	
duck, moose			green apples	peanuts	
lamb			pears	almonds	
salmon	nuts / seeds			pecans	
turkey, dark meat	all okay			other nuts	
wild game	legumes		legumes		
eggs	low-starch		low-starch		

Mixed Type

Mixed Types are a combination of the Carb Type and Protein Type and should obtain an equal mix of the Carb Type and Protein Type recommendations. For example, Mixed Types should obtain a balance between the high-purine meats from the Protein Type Recommended Foods Table and the low-purine, low-fat proteins from the Carb Type Recommended Foods Table. In addition, Mixed Types also need to pay careful attention to how foods make them feel to make the necessary adjustments. If you are possibly a Mixed Type based on the test earlier in this chapter, it is again highly recommended you take the more comprehensive start in William Wolcott's *The Metabolic Typing Diet* book to help you hone in more reliably, but you can start now by taking a mixed approach to all the guidelines for both the Carb and Protein Types above, listening to your body after eating, and fine-tuning in the direction that is best for you. For instance, start by eating about an equal amount of lighter meats like chicken and turkey breast and darker meats like grass-fed beef and bison. Assess which generally make you feel better between and hour and three hours after eating and edge your diet in the direction of eating more of those meats. The same goes for the vegetables, fruits, oils, nuts, etc. defined above. In general you'll always be able to eat some amount of all the types of foods; by listening to your body and fine-tuning you'll soon be able to determine if you edge more in the direction of a Carb or Protein Type.

6: Overcoming Emotional Barriers, Nourishing the Mind and Spirit

There is no separating mental health from physical health. You cannot truly have one without the other. The wonderful thing is, as you improve your physical health you will improve mental health and vice versa. By following the dietary recommendations in this book, you will prevent and fight disease, optimize weight, have a youthful appearance and increase your physical strength, and you'll also be nourishing your nervous system for optimal mental functioning. The reverse is also true. By addressing your mental issues and removing the emotional obstacles to cure, you can greatly improve your physical health.

The reason why we have such incredible results with our patients at the Optimal Wellness Center is that we take great care to address the whole person—mind, body and spirit. For example, if a patient with arthritis has a great deal of anxiety, following the perfect diet still may not help if they do not address their anxiety problem. Both areas need to be healed to have real and permanent success. In all people, without exception, there are both mental and physical issues that hold them back from being in perfect health. That is why this next section is vitally important.

How to Overcome Emotional Barriers

You now know one of the most important steps you can take to prevent disease and optimize weight is to eliminate processed grains and sugars from your diet. "But wait," some of you may think, "that means no more loaves of French bread. No more English muffins or bagels. No more cakes, pies, and cookies. I don't think I can do that." That type of thinking is an emotional barrier. For some, there is the demon of self-doubt and resistance lurking inside you and, even though you know this crucial step would benefit your health, your self-doubt makes you feel like you couldn't possibly succeed. So where did that little demon come from, and why does it seem in control of you?

You may think you lack willpower if you have cravings for and addictions to food, but that is not true. It's not that you lack willpower, but that you never learned the tools for how to address your addictions and emotional challenges. In my clinical practice, attending to emotional issues is central to the program. The majority of these emotional barriers can be traced back to childhood. For instance, in our society we reward children by giving them junk food such as birthday cakes, cupcakes, ice cream or McDonald's Happy Meals. In addition, children are inundated by junk food marketing on TV. This emotional patterning remains with them into adulthood, and so it may initially seem "impossible" to some to abandon processed grains and sweets. Other common emotional blocks leading to self-defeating behaviors include deep-seated traumas such as abuse, low self-esteem, chronic high stress, depression and anxiety, dysfunctional childhood, mimicking behaviors of parents, and self-medicating with food.

Over the years, my clinical staff and I have researched and practiced a wide variety of therapeutic methods to address these blocks. The technique that we have had the greatest success with is called Emotional Freedom Technique, or EFT, and it is remarkably easy to learn and do. When people do EFT for the first time they are, though, sometimes a bit skeptical. At first glance it may look strange as it involves tapping on specific acupuncture points while speaking affirmations of self-acceptance aloud to acknowledge the issue at hand. But EFT really works because it heals disruptions in the body's energy system. Everything we see, hear, feel, taste, and smell is transmitted along our nerves to our brain through electrochemical messages in our energy system. If you touch a hot stove, you feel pain due to the nerve endings in your hand sending instantaneous electrochemical messages through your nerves to your brain. Our body's electrical system is essential to our physical health and without it we die.

The electrical system of our body has been known about since the Chinese, 5,000 years ago, discovered channels of energy flowing through the body. Chinese medicine refers to these channels as meridians, and the energy that flows through them is called "Qi," pronounced "chi." The Chinese discovered that by superficially inserting tiny needles into specific acupuncture points on the skin, they were able to release blocked energy in the meridians and therefore restore a person back to equilibrium.

EFT works in a similar manner; instead of using needles, EFT is performed by tapping with fingers on acupuncture points at the end of the meridians. As people tap on these points, they tune into their emotional problem by repeating affirmations about the problem such as, "Even though I eat junk food to help me cope with stress, I deeply and completely accept myself." Effective affirmations follow the same general format—they acknowledge the problem and create self-acceptance despite the existence of the problem.

EFT is based on the premise that the cause of all negative emotions is a disruption in the body's energy system. When a person experiences an emotional trauma, the intense emotion causes a short-circuit somewhere in the electrical system of the body. Picture what would happen to the television screen of a show you are watching if you went behind the set and started to pull the wires apart. The picture would eventually turn snowy because you short-circuited the TV. The snowy picture is an analogy for a negative emotion. The same effect occurs when you experience negative emotions—there is a short circuit somewhere in your body's energy system. By tuning into the problem and tapping on multiple points, EFT stimulates the meridians, sending pulses of energy down the channels that heal the negative emotions that are blocking the energy flow in the channels. The most common responses people have after doing EFT are an elimination of pain, a feeling of peace and relaxation, and a feeling that their unwanted negative emotion no longer affects them.

While it is easy to learn, though, the one drawback with the Emotional Freedom Technique is that it can't be easily learned by reading about it. On Mercola.com for a time, and in various publications, the attempt was made to provide a "how-to do EFT" in the two-dimensional form of screens and pages, but it's something like learning the right golf swings from a page: not very effective. We found that people frequently did not understand how to use the affirmations.

Therefore, while you will find it is easy to learn and use once you see it, it is highly recommended that you learn from a source where you can see it in action. The best options for learning doing so are either with a trained EFT therapist or a live seminar or video training course. To find a qualified EFT therapist in your area, go to the Mercola.com homepage and at the bottom click on "Find a Health Practitioner in Your Area." To locate EFT seminar information, you can enter the keyword "EFT" on Google.com. The most inexpensive option is to watch my six-hour EFT Training Course, available on DVD or VHS. This course can be ordered from the Mercola.com homepage under the "Recommended Products" section. In this video course, I teach you step-by-step all the information you need to use EFT for your emotional healing. I provide live demonstrations of EFT with real people and show how long-standing emotional issues can disappear within minutes with this wonderful tool. For those who are skeptical and think this sounds too good to be true, the EFT Training Course comes with a full 12-month money back guarantee.

EFT is not the only way to overcome emotional barriers. Conventional one-on-one therapy, acupuncture, group therapy and a host of other approaches have certainly helped people. I have also heard that many people have experienced success with The Sedona Method, which is available in an audio program by that name by Hale Dwoskin, and it may be worth your while to explore it as well. But overall, EFT has definitely proven to be one of the most effective ways. If you find yourself confronting cravings, addictions, depression, self-image issues or other barriers to implementing a healthy diet and lifestyle, though, don't let those barriers hold you back: seek some form of therapy as soon as possible as it is fundamental to reaching your ideal health.

Feeding Your Mind and Spirit

In addition to healing the physical and emotional body, total health also means nourishing the spirit. The spirit is an essential part of the mind-body-spirit triumvirate that is rarely addressed in medicine. Most spiritual experts agree that the two most powerful methods of evolving one's spirituality are prayer and meditation. While prayer is an act of communion with and devotion to God, it has been shown in numerous studies to have a very positive influence on physical health. Meditation is a part of many spiritual disciplines but is also used as a means of quieting the mind to bring about a deep healing relaxation response in the body. Meditation was one of multiple therapies Dr. Dean Ornish successfully employed in his famous clinical trials using natural methods for reversing heart disease. In study after study, meditation has proven to have a direct and very positive influence on physical health. In one study published in the British Medical Journal in 2001, for instance, forms of meditation such as saying the Rosary and reciting a mantra from Yoga were found to have a very positive effect on the respiratory system and heart. It has also been shown to lead to improved digestion and immunity, and therefore disease prevention.

If you are interested in learning more about all the studies demonstrating the link between prayer, meditation and health, you can enter those terms into the search engine at Mercola.com. *Healing Words*, a classic book by Larry Dossey who has written extensively on the effects of prayer on health, is also a very worthwhile read.

If you want to learn meditation there are many approaches available. Some of these, like forms of Yoga, Tai Chi and Chi Kung (also known as "Qigong"), are a meditation in motion by slowly performing low-impact movements to strengthen the body and calm the mind. When most people think of meditation they imagine sitting cross-legged with closed eyes while chanting "Om." This is only one form of meditation among thousands that you could learn. However, the basic principle is the same: the goal of meditation is to quiet the mind, to access the "gap" or the place of no thoughts, to commune with one's soul and with God. The basic practice is to sit upright, close your eyes and focus on the breath. Reciting a word such as peace or love may help in focusing. Anytime a thought enters your mind, gently brush it aside and go back to the breath. The optimal amount of time to meditate is 20 minutes in the morning and in the evening.

In addition to the powerful health benefits of prayer and meditation, always remember that any experience that positively engages your mind and warms your heart is very good for your over-all health. Activities such as reading, for instance, have proven health benefits. This means not only reading books like this one, which provide you with practical steps to take toward health, but also reading stories and spiritual works that can expand your consciousness. When people read a quality novel or spiritual book, they often feel a sense of elation that is indeed good for your overall health. That's why listening to your favorite music, going to art shows, and other such acts that engage the mind and heart and produce a similar uplifting feeling are more than just entertainment—they feel good because they are good for you. They actually generate a variety of neuropeptides and hormones in your brain that can improve your health. The same goes for taking walks with a loved one, playing games with children, pursuing hobbies and interests as a group, and any of the end-less social activities available to us. We're social beings, and engaging in positive acts together is absolutely critical to nurturing your mind, spirit and body. Best of all, they are enjoyable. Really living life, to conclude, is one of the most important steps you can take to live longer.

7: Four Lifestyle Factors For Total Health

Healthy Water... Drink Up!

Drinking eight glasses a day of pure water is an important foundational health principle for most people. An alarming number of Americans don't follow this guideline and are constantly dehydrated. Dehydration is subtle and most don't feel the thirst on their tongue, but their bodies are suffering—without sufficient water intake they cannot properly detoxify and aid their bodies in the elimination of wastes. Some minor symptoms of insufficient water intake are headaches, feeling tired and groggy, constipation and dry skin. If left untended, dehydration can contribute to a variety of serious health problems with blood pressure, circulation, kidney function, immune system function, and digestive disorders.

For many people, I recommend drinking one quart of water for every fifty pounds of body weight per day, but keep in mind this may be too much water for some people. A simple test for determining if you are drinking enough water is to watch the color of your urine over a period of several days. It should be very lightly colored. If it is darker in color it is concentrated and you would likely benefit from increasing your water intake. Note, though, that if you are taking vitamin B2 (riboflavin), either by itself or in a multi-vitamin, it will turn urine bright yellow and you will not be able to use this self-test. Discontinue the vitamin for 24 hours while maintaining your normal water drinking levels to properly determine if you need more water in your diet.

As with each type of food, the form and source of your water are vital to your health. Just because water is listed as potable does not mean it is good for you. In general, tap water should be avoided because it contains chlorine and usually fluoride, both toxic substances that can have dire consequences for your body over time. Many people are surprised to hear that fluoride in tap water is not good, as municipalities starting adding it to water based on research from fifty years ago to "help our teeth." Since that time, though, studies have shown, and experts have come forth to testify, that the risks of fluoride far outweigh any benefit. Fluoride is more toxic than lead and is used as a pesticide for mice, rats and other small pests. The fluoride used in tap water is not closely monitored (and is even considered an "unapproved drug" by the FDA), and often contains high levels of carcinogens like arsenic. Indeed, fluoride has been directly linked to cancer and to weakened bones and osteoporosis; you can read much more about all the studies proving the dangers of the fluoridation of tap water by typing in "fluoride" on Mercola.com's search engine. Beyond chlorine and fluoride, though, there are still many other reasons to be cautious of tap water. At water treatment facilities, water is inundated with other chemicals including algaecides, oxidants, and pH inhibitors, and the effect of these chemicals is not entirely known on the human body. Furthermore, in many municipalities, particularly those in and around big cities, the water then runs through pipes that can be decades or even over a hundred years old, and then enters pipes in homes that may be corroded or welded using lead materials. Tap water health risks are also a problem with cooking, as the toxic substances are absorbed in the food, and with showering, as your body absorbs chlorine and other toxic substances through the skin.

To ensure the safety of the water out of your tap, you should first have it evaluated and tested. You can check your phonebook or call your town's chamber of commerce to locate a service that can do this, but for a higher level of assurance I recommend you contact an EPA-certified laboratory to test your water. If you have any problem finding such a service, there is a free home water evaluation available from the Water Safety Council through Mercola.com in the "Recommended Products" section that will provide information on how your municipal water is rated. The Water Safety Council also offers a series of EPA-certified water tests you can perform on your own by mailing in vials of your water for a nominal fee. If you know your home water supply is high in specific contaminants, you can appropriately choose a water filtration system designed to eliminate those particular contaminants. This is important, as there are many filtration systems on the market but not all are designed to eliminate all contaminants. To remove fluoride, I recommend a reverse osmosis filter. Carbon-based filters are generally economical, but if you choose to use them instead of a reverse osmosis filter, more expensive carbon matrix inserts are required to remove fluoride.

Drinking distilled water should also be avoided; distilled water is, first of all, highly acidic. Most people are far too acidic already and more acid will continue to push the PH of the body in the wrong direction. And though distilled water is supposed to be free of contaminants, many of the devices that distill the water are made of metal and actually add certain toxic metals like nickel into the water. Another important point is that distilled water has an osmotic gradient because it is a hypotonic solution. If a hypotonic solution (low in particles) interacts with another solution that is hypertonic (high in particles, such as the bloodstream) then the particles will gravitate from the high to the low solution. This means that distilled water can actually leach beneficial minerals out of your bloodstream and out of your body. While some people have claimed distilled water provides detoxification over the short term because of this, over the long run this is highly counterproductive. Water also has a very delicate atomic structure that can be easily damaged when it is mechanically distilled.

In addition to properly filtered tap water, bottled spring water is another option. It is not my first choice though as the energy involved in transporting the water and in making the plastic disposable bottles poses quite a significant burden on the environment. If you use spring (not "drinking") water it should be bottled in clear polyethylene or glass containers, not the one-gallon plastic (PVC) containers that will leach plastic chemicals into the water. Also be careful that the water comes from a real spring, as about forty percent of the bottled waters on the market are not from a spring but a tap (including popular brands like Aquafina and Dasani.) Read the labels carefully. As the price of one bottle of Evian can equal what you'd pay for 1000 gallons of home tap water, though, your most economical choice is definitely to have your tap water professionally tested and to invest in an appropriate filtration system.

Fall Madly In Love... With Exercise

You've heard it a million times, and every time you hear it you're hearing the truth: you need to exercise. Exercise is essential to my Total Health Program, and should be as high a priority in your life as proper eating and sleeping. Here's the first rule of thumb to remember—find the forms of exercise you enjoy and do those. With so many options available, there's no need to force yourself to do activities you hate. You are far more likely to succeed at something you enjoy. The second rule of thumb is this—no matter what your age, no matter what your current health condition, there's always a higher level of physical health to reach for, which is really a main purpose of life— to constantly strive to grow and improve. Exercise is not a temporary pursuit to attain a certain waist size or biceps width but a lifelong habit that, if pursued properly, will increase the quality and length of your life. It in addition to helping you look and feel younger, it will improve your body's ability to fight and prevent disease, increase your brain functioning and energy, decrease depression, and help you sleep better. Pair it with proper diet and emotional health as outlined in this book and you will feel the way you are designed to be, always full of energy and joy.

Where to Start if You Haven't Been Exercising

If you are over age 35 and have not exercised in years, or if you have a health problem, it is important to consult with your physician before exercising. Ask your physician if there are specific exercises you should avoid or focus on for your condition.

Start your exercise regime in "manageable bites" and gradually increase. Particularly with exercise, people have a tendency to overdo it from the start because they are charged with motivation; you can achieve the body of an athlete, but if you start off with a workout routine akin to an athlete, you're bound to injure yourself and give up because of the difficulty. Remind yourself to progress slowly, little step by little step. Another key point is to always listen to your body. If some form of exercise seems to be worsening your symptoms, you will need to modify your program. If the pain or discomfort continues with exercise, stop and consult with your physician.

You can start your workout regime by doing low-impact exercise that works both your heart and muscles about thirty minutes per day. If you are confined indoors, elliptical machines provide an exceptional low-impact total-body workout. But if you can head outdoors, walking is a wonderful exercise to begin with. Walking is very low-impact so it's easy on the joints and it requires little equipment except a good pair of walking shoes. Furthermore, it's a great opportunity to see the world around you, be out in the sun, and clear your head. It is helpful to do some light stretching before you exercise. Begin either at a slow pace and gradually increase to a pace that elevates your heart rate and is intense enough that it is difficult to carry on a conversation. In the final few minutes decrease the pace of your workout to cool down. Please remember that in order to continually improve your cardiovascular fitness levels you need to increase the intensity over time.

Increase the Intensity & Include Weight Training

Once you're in the habit of exercising, you should increase your workout time to sixty minutes per day. If you need to lose weight, you should workout five to seven days per week, but once you are in shape and at your ideal weight three or four times a week is sufficient. Ideally, the exercise should be continuous, but with people's busy schedules it can be split up into two thirty-minute routines.

Running is an outstanding weight-bearing exercise, and weight-bearing exercises are especially helpful for prevention of osteoporosis. I have been running since 1968, and while I've tried many other exercises, I've found it's one of the most efficient and inexpensive ways to stay in shape. Contrary to popular belief, running is not harmful to your knees if you have high-quality running shoes. Also remember to change your running shoes about once every six months in order to avoid injury. There are of course countless other ways out there to get exercise. Swimming is quite good, but the challenge is that swimming pools contain large amounts of chlorine that is absorbed into the skin, so it is better if you can swim in a lake, river or ocean. Sports like basketball, tennis and the martial arts also provide first-rate workouts, but are higher-impact and therefore more prone to injury.

For indoor workouts or for those who need to maintain a low-impact workout, elliptical machines are an outstanding choice. Their oval-shaped pedaling motion is far easier on the joints than treadmills and other equipment, and ellipticals provide both excellent weight-bearing and cardiovascular benefits. Walking or race walking is another great option for many.

Finally, everyone should also incorporate weight training into his or her exercise regime. Weight training is a great way to tone muscles, increase bone density, and burn fat and calories throughout the day. When you begin weight training, you should either consider hiring a personal trainer (you don't have to pay megabucks, as most park districts have them on-staff), or invest in a reputable book or video guide to weight training and follow all of the precautionary advice and steps for each type of weight exercise carefully. There are various approaches to weight training, from circuit training (a series of resistance exercises performed one after another with little rest between exercises) to the conventional moderately paced sets (a minute of rest in between each set) to the SuperSlow workouts where weights are lifted and lowered at a very slow pace. I have personally utilized the SuperSlow method (through the guidance of a personal trainer) and achieved greater benefit with it in shorter time than the conventional method. It requires less time than a conventional weight-training program, but be warned that it is also a more strenuous workout. Regardless of the style of weight lifting you choose, you will want to radically change your routine each month in order to prevent your muscles from adapting to the workout and causing a plateau.

22 Ways To Sleep Well

Many people do not realize just how important proper sleep is for their health. With today's hectic lifestyle, our society is sleeping less in order to work more. Research studies show that depriving the sleep your body needs decreases the quality of your life and decreases your longevity. Inadequate sleep disrupts health in many ways such as leading to hormonal and metabolism imbalances, accelerated aging, increased onset and severity of type-2 diabetes, high blood pressure, obesity, memory loss, and more. Insomnia is an epidemic as 25% of Americans have occasional insomnia and 10% have chronic insomnia. Here are some helpful guidelines to improve the quality of your sleep, and therefore your health:

1) For most people, seven to nine hours is an ideal amount of sleep, with more people requiring nine hours versus seven.

2)   You should try to get to bed before 11 p.m. Your body performs the majority of its repair and recovery functions during the hours of 11 p.m. and 1 a.m. For example, the gallbladder dumps toxins during this period. If you are awake, the toxins back up into the liver, which then sends toxins into your bloodstream. It is interesting to note that prior to electricity, people went to bed at sundown as they followed their instinctual biorhythms to arise and retire by the sun.

3)   Seek to go to bed and wake up at the same times each day, even on weekends. This will help your body to get into a sleep rhythm and make it easier to fall asleep and get up in the morning.

4)   Sleep in complete darkness or as close to it as possible. When light hits the eyes, it disrupts the circadian rhythm of the pineal gland and production of melatonin and serotonin, disrupting the quality of sleep. You can achieve this with blackout blinds, shades or draperies over the bedroom windows, or with a sleep mask covering the eyes.

5)   Avoid eating right before bedtime as the digestive process can impair sleep. Moreover, eating grains and sugars can cause an eventual hypoglycemia (low blood sugar), which can cause hunger and sleep disturbance.

6)   Avoid T.V. before bed. Even better, remove the T.V. from the bedroom. T.V. is stimulating to the brain, which disrupts the pineal gland, making it harder to fall asleep or sleep well. The same holds true for avoidance of reading materials that you find stimulating. If you read before bed, opt to read books that are relaxing and peaceful such as spiritual literature.

7)   Wear socks to bed. Due to the fact that feet have the poorest circulation, they tend to feel cold before the rest of the body, which can disrupt your sleep.

8)   Avoid using loud alarm clocks. It is very stressful on the body to awaken with a sudden loud noise. Ideally, you should sleep until your body naturally awakens, making an alarm clock unnecessary. If you need an alarm, use a dawn simulator, which gradually emits light to full intensity over 45 minutes, much like the morning sun. It is a gentle awakening that doesn't startle the adrenals that would begin your day in fight or flight mode. Type in the words "dawn simulator" on Google.com for the retailers who sell them.

9)   Before bed, turn the alarm clock face down so you are unable to see the time. If you have trouble falling asleep, it will only provoke worry and keep you awake when you keep staring at the time.

10) If you lie in bed with your mind racing, it might be helpful to keep a journal and write down your thoughts before bed. This achieves the effect of downloading your disturbing thoughts to paper to clear your mind.

11) Keep the temperature in the bedroom 60–70 degrees F, as anything warmer can disrupt sleep.

12) Eat a high-protein snack, such as grass-fed beef jerky, several hours before bed. This can provide the L-tryptophan need to produce melatonin and serotonin. Also eat a small piece of fruit or a handful of berries around the same time. This can help the tryptophan cross the blood-brain barrier.

13) Consider that both prescription and over-the-counter drugs may have negative effects on sleep. Keep your drug use to only what is absolutely necessary.

14) Avoid caffeine and other stimulants, as they can have long lasting stimulatory effects on the nervous system. Note that some medications, such as over-the-counter pain relievers (e.g. Midol) and diet pills, contain caffeine.

15) Avoid alcohol. Although alcohol will make people drowsy, the effect is short-lived and people will often wake up several hours later, unable to fall back asleep. Alcohol will also keep you from falling into the deeper stages of REM sleep, where the body does most of its healing.

16) Avoid foods to which you are sensitive. This is particularly true for dairy and wheat products, as they may have a negative effect on sleep, such as causing apnea, excess congestion, gastrointestinal upset, and gas.

17) If you tend to wake up at night to urinate, don't drink any fluids within 2 hours of going to bed.

18) Take a hot bath, shower or sauna for about 30 to 60 minutes before bed. Heat has a relaxing effect on the body.

19) Don't do work in your bed or bedroom. If you do, you may find it is harder to disassociate from work activities when trying to fall asleep.

20) Exercise helps to burn off stress and clear the mind, but as exercise energizes the body, don't exercise too close to bedtime.

21) Listen to white noise or relaxation CDs. Some people find the sound of white noise or nature sounds, such as rainfall or ocean waves, soothing for sleep.

22) Sleep in a comfortable bed. If your mattress is sagging, makes creaking noises, or if you wake up with stiffness or back pain, it may be time for a new mattress. Chiropractors can be a resource for helping you determine the type of mattress you should sleep on. Avoid waterbeds, as they do not properly support the spine.

Supplements: Don't Overdo Them, But Do Consider These

A majority of Americans, Canadians, Australians, and Europeans take some form of nutritional supplementation, and therefore the supplement business is a multi-billion dollar industry. Yet, most supplements are unnecessary if people eat a healthy diet. Eat a mediocre or poor diet and you can supplement until your bank account is dry, but you still won't be making a positive dent in improving your health. Vegetables, naturally raised meats and other good foods contain not only the vitamins you need, but also a long and complex list of micronutrients that cannot be found in any supplement.

That said, there are a few supplements that everyone should consider taking. As you'll see, most of these are not "supplements" in the conventional sense of the word, since they are actually real foods. Remember that if you have a negative reaction to any food or supplement, discontinue it. Your body will tell you what it does or does not need.

Fish Oil/Cod Liver Oil for Essential Omega-3

Most people are seriously lacking essential omega-3 fatty acids in their diet. In fact, while the ideal ratio of omega-6 to omega-3 should be 1:1, the typical American—on a diet high in corn, soy, canola and other unsaturated oils, corn-fed beef, etc.—has a ratio ranging from 20:1 to 50:1! That alone is a prescription for a major health disaster.

Omega-3 fatty acids are essential fatty acids (EFA). This means that they are essential for life but that the body does not make them and it therefore must obtain them from the diet. Omega-3 fats are pivotal for energy production, oxygen transfer, hemoglobin production, membrane components, muscle recovery, prostaglandin (hormone like substances) production, growth, and cell division, immune function and brain development. Omega-3 fats also help produce soft smooth skin, and increase healing, vitality, and calmness. Furthermore, omega-3 fats reduce inflammation, water retention, platelet stickiness, blood pressure, and tumor growth.

The omega-3 family consists of: 1) Alpha-Linolenic Acid (ALA), which is found in flax, hemp seed, canola, soy bean, walnut, and dark-green leaves; and 2) EPA and DHA, which is found in oils of cold water fish such as salmon, trout, mackerel, sardines and marine animals. DHA and EPA from fish oil is the best source of omega-3 fats because the body can directly use this DHA and EPA for its numerous functions. On the other hand, ALA have to undergo a series of biochemical conversions to result in DHA and EPA, and most people lack the enzymes to make these conversions as these enzymes are damaged by improper nutrition and stress.

Unfortunately, as covered in Chapter 4, virtually all fish are contaminated with mercury and other dangerous industrial toxins, thus the risks of eating polluted fish far outweigh the omega-3 benefits. If you are a Protein Metabolic Type in particular, you would be doing your body much good in terms of protein and this omega-3 by eating fish that has been lab-tested and shown not to contain these harmful toxins. If you are unable to locate any in your local markets that you are certain are free of harmful mercury and PCBs, you can find toxin-free wild red Alaskan salmon through the "Recommended Products" section of Mercola.com.

Due to the fact that 95% of Americans are deficient in omega-3 fatty acids, everyone needs to take fish oil or cod liver oil. Most Americans are so deficient in omega-3 fats, it would take consuming 12 bottles of omega-3 oil over a period of months for the average American to attain normal omega-3 levels and to maintain normal levels; therefore, it is highly recommended to take omega-3 oils on a daily basis for life.

There are a few important points to consider when choosing fish oil or cod liver oil. These oils are very perishable and fragile and can easily oxidize; for that reason and more, quality assurance is an extremely important issue with fish and cod liver oil. There is a great difference in the quality from one brand to the next due to the manufacturing processes used, the source of the fish and more. After carefully reviewing cod liver oils and fish oils over the years, including what processes should be used in their creation, I most highly recommend Garden of Life's "Olde World Icelandic Cod Liver Oil" and Living Fuel's "Omega 3 & E" fish oil capsules. The Carlson's brand of fish oil is also recommended. These brands contain no trace of toxins or heavy metals and had very low levels of oxidized fats. Garden of Life's cod liver oil is exceptionally pure and is made with very minimal processing. Living Fuel's fish oil capsules, meanwhile, contain tocotrienols and tocopherols, which as you will read in "Vitamin E" below means you are getting the necessary vitamin E right in the same capsule. You can find these brands of fish and cod liver oils at some health food stores, and they are also available through the "Recommended Products" section of Mercola.com.

As a rule of thumb, you should take fish oil during the months that you spend time in the sun, and take cod liver oil in the cooler to cold-weather months. Even if it is sunny and warm, there is not enough UVB radiation present to cause your body to make enough vitamin D in the winter. Cod liver oil, unlike fish oil, provides the extra benefit of being high in vitamin D. On a side note, I perform vitamin D testing on all my patients since vitamin D deficiency is widespread and a major contributor to the cancer epidemic. Among other benefits, vitamin D aids in the absorption of calcium. (If you have any concerns about your vitamin D level, you should have your vitamin D level tested, as high levels can lead to osteoporosis and hardening of your arteries. Many health care practitioners will not be aware of the importance of vitamin D testing, so feel free to search for more on this important topic on Mercola.com, and watch the Mercola newsletter for a forthcoming national resource that can perform this testing and more for you.)

The recommended daily adult dose of fish oil or cod liver oil is one teaspoon. Children should take one ml for every ten pounds of body weight up to a maximum of one teaspoon.

Full-Spectrum Vitamin E

Vitamin E is an excellent anti-oxidant that protects cell membranes, defends fatty acids from oxidative damage, decreases inflammation, assists with nerve and muscle function, and helps prevent cancer and heart disease. It is especially useful if you are taking fish oils. It is important to read the labels on vitamin E bottles, as you want to take vitamin E that lists "tocopherols and tocotrienols" to obtain the full spectrum of biological activity. Avoid labels that list "dl-alpha-tocopherol," which is the synthetic form of vitamin E and grossly inferior to the natural form. Unfortunately, most of the vitamin E on grocery store shelves is synthetic because it is cheaper to produce, but you should be able to find full-spectrum vitamin E in most health food stores. For adults, I recommend taking 400 IU of vitamin E daily.

Anyone that is not consuming large amounts of vegetables like dark leafy greens (turnip, mustard and collard greens, kale, chard, lettuce, spinach), green tea, broccoli, and cabbage on a daily basis would likely benefit from supplementing with vitamin K. Also, it is important for women with a family history of osteoporosis or women with risk factors for osteoporosis to supplement with vitamin K. In Japan, vitamin K is the treatment of choice for osteoporosis.

Vitamin K has been shown to:
- Both prevent and treat cancer
- Build strong bones and prevent osteoporosis, serving as biological bone "glue" that carries calcium into the bone matrix
- Aid in preventing hardening of the arteries and avoiding coronary artery disease and heart attacks

I advise using vitamin K1, a natural plant-based vitamin K, or K2, a bacterially based vitamin K, versus the synthetic K3. I suggest a starting dose of 3000 mcg of vitamin K1 or K2 per day. Since the body does not easily absorb vitamin K, it should be taken with meals that include fat to increase absorption.

Probiotics to Build Your Immunity

There are 100 trillion bacteria, weighing a total of three pounds, lining your intestinal tract. This complex system of beneficial bacteria is a crucial part of your immune system, protecting your body from invasions. However, they are not an infallible army: the "Standard American Diet" (SAD for short) is high in sugar, processed food and toxic chemicals that feeds the pathogenic gut bacteria and depletes the beneficial bacteria. The lack of a fully effective army of good bacteria in your gut will impair your immune system and can predispose you to many types of illness.

To maintain the good bacteria, the most important thing you should do is adopt the diet outlined in this book, including eating the clean and healthy types of foods discussed. Second, and especially if you are not eating fermented foods containing good bacteria daily (e.g. kefir, sauerkraut, kimchee, etc), you should supplement with a high-quality "probiotic," or good bacteria. Probiotics are active bacterial cultures like lactobacillus, acidophilus, and bifudis, but be careful as many of the products labeled "probiotic" have been found to contain no living bacteria whatsoever, or not all of the types listed on the label. I have researched and experimented with numerous brands of probiotics, and I've had the best results with the "Primal Defense" brand of probiotics. You can order Primal Defense through Mercola.com or you can find it at your local health products store.

It is best to take your probiotics with food. If you are traveling to a foreign country, it is also a good idea to take probiotics with you. In the event you get infectious traveler's diarrhea, large doses of a high-quality probiotics—one-half to a full bottle per day—can clear the diarrhea within hours.

Chlorella, the Heavy Metal Magnet

Chlorella is a single-cell marine alga available in capsule, tablet or granule format, and it is a superb supplement to anyone's diet. Chlorella, while newer to the West, is the most popular supplement in Japan because it is considered a "miracle food." It affords an unsurpassed ability to detoxify the heavy metals and other contaminants from the body, and is also an effective antibiotic and antiviral. Further, it helps to cleanse the bowels, aids in the production of beneficial bacteria, and in the production of red blood cells. Meanwhile, it contains a high amount of vitamin B12, minerals and protein, which makes it a noteworthy supplement for vegetarians. Also, the vitamins and minerals in chlorella are bio-chelated, which means they are naturally wrapped in amino acids so the body will more readily take them in than store-bought vitamins.

You do, however, need to be very careful about the quality of chlorella you choose, as it should be raised in pure waters and packaged while still fresh. The chlorella I highly recommend is produced by Yaeyama, a company with over 35 years experience in chlorella research, and known worldwide for its high quality and absolute purity. Their chlorella is ecologically grown in mineral-rich mountain spring water in the pure air and sunshine, without any pesticides. Potency and purity meet the most rigorous Japanese health standards, and it contains no sugar, starch, or artificial coloring, flavoring or preservatives. You can find Yaeyama chlorella on Mercola.com in the "Recommended Products" section.

As chlorella is a whole food, it is highly perishable, so I strongly urge you to make sure that your chlorella is packaged in opaque plastic bottles that are made from P.T.E. plastic and contain ultraviolet inhibitors; this prevents U.V. rays from penetrating and damaging the chlorella quality. You should also ensure that the package seal is airtight after every use to that no air penetrates the chlorella and damages its fragile micronutrients.

I recommend about three (3) grams of chlorella daily to benefit from its nutritional properties.

Healthy Meal Replacements

The recipes in this book were created with ease of preparation in mind, but the reality is that in today's busy world, you don't always have time to make a meal. For example, when traveling, many people break from their healthy diet because they are not able to prepare their own meals, and they grab a corn-fed burger with a side of trans-fat fries and a sugar-laced Coke instead. Problem is, this is one of the most common situations in which successful diets break apart. One bad meal turns to two, two turns to four, and before they realize it, people are back to old bad habits.

If you suspect that you won't have time to prepare a healthy meal, the smartest approach is to be prepared with a high-quality "superfood" meal replacement. I'm not talking about energy bars that tend to provide little real nutritional value in relation to their sugars, carbohydrates and calories, but a nutritious meal replacement made from whole foods and freeze-dried for easy mixture in water. There are a variety of them available, and while none provide the nutrition that a meal containing fresh and healthy foods fit for your metabolic type can, some are far better options than fast food, convenience store snacks, or meals at places like Denny's.

Because many of my patients often travel, and because I often do as well, I have researched and tried many of these meal replacements. By far the best one I have found is called Living Fuel.

It's made of all-natural food products that provide a wide range of nutrients and contains no genetically modified organisms, pesticides, herbicides, or other chemicals. You simply mix it with water, so it's also easy to use. Some of my patients take Living Fuel as a daily nutritional supplement while others use it as a meal-on-the-run when they are pressed for time. If you can't find it in your local health food store, you can find out more about it in the "Recommended Products" section on Mercola.com. Whatever brand of convenience "superfood" you choose, remember that they're excellent as back-up meals, but nothing can replace the nutritional value of healthy meats, vegetables, and all the other foods previously discussed.

A Supplemental Recommendation on Supplements

I am known as a minimalist when it comes to supplements, but what that means should be clear: I advocate eating the proper foods in the appropriate proportions to your needs as the primary means to your vibrant health and wellness. It bears repeating that nothing—absolutely nothing—is as crucial to fighting disease and premature aging, increasing your energy, prolonging your life, and of course optimizing your weight as healthy eating.

One of the major issues with supplements is that many people, brainwashed by the pharmaceutical culture to believe that a pill—or handfuls of them—can somehow "fix" their broken health, are blindly opting for handfuls of supplements, somehow believing these endless vitamin supplements are somehow more "natural" and "wholesome" than pharmaceutical drugs, and therefore the right thing to do. Meanwhile, they have forgotten the inherent definition of "supplement"—that is, an addition that compensates for a missing piece in something that is otherwise good—and are instead using supplements as the magical medicinal main act. I have seen many a new patient walk into my clinic showing me bagfuls of supplements they've been taking who are astonished at their horrid and declining health and begging me to tell them "what supplements are missing?"

Ninety-nine times out of a hundred it's not that "some" supplement is missing, though. It's that they're totally ignoring or misguided on the real main act—their diet. They may down fifteen different supplements every morning, but then they head off to a day of meals that includes processed grains, added sugars, grain-fed beef and farm-raised fish, trans-fats, and artificially sweetened sodas. Their diet is defeating their health and immune system, and no supplement will help them. Worse, that same ninety-nine times out of a hundred, all of the supplements they are taking are actually making things worse. That's because of the other major issue with supplements: quality, or the lack thereof.

The quality of supplements, like the quality of your food, means everything in terms of its benefits to your health. For example, the synthetic form of vitamin E, d,l-alpha tocopherol, is cheap to produce and therefore that is the form you will find on most grocery store shelves. The problem with synthetic vitamin E is that it is only half as bio-available to the body as the natural form of vitamin E d-alpha tocopheryl. Most manufacturers know that the mass public is not aware of these major differences in the quality of ingredients and therefore chooses the cheapest ingredients possible to increase profitability at the sacrifice of your health. Because of this issue, if you are taking low-quality supplements you are probably better off taking none at all, as is it could be doing more harm than good. I have reviewed the clinical benefits of a wide variety of supplements for many years, and while there are certainly other companies out there with high-quality products, there are a few companies whose supplement products I have personally come to trust: Garden of Life, Living Fuel, and Biotics. This is not a blanket endorsement for every single supplement they offer, as 1) I have not reviewed every single supplement they each offer and 2) I don't want to give you the misimpression that I recommend bagfuls of supplements when instead I urge you to first and foremost focus on your diet. But because of their focus on the highest-quality ingredients and processes, these are some of the companies I recommend you consider if there is a specific supplement you are certain you require beyond those I covered above.

On a final note, there are possibly a few other supplements you may want to consider depending on your particular health challenges and where you are on your journey to optimal wellness. For instance, through my routine vitamin D testing some of my patients show severe vitamin D deficiency and require more than the supplemental cod liver oil mentioned above; I recommend Biotics vitamin D. My ultimate point is that some supplements are beneficial to take if you remember what "supplemental" means, and if you remain vigilant about consuming only the highest quality.

8: Pulling It All Together: Your Personal Total Health Plan

You've come this far, and you now have over two decades of my own professional experience. Congratulations! Perhaps you're a bit overwhelmed with exactly what to do with it all. Therefore, this section has been designed to help you pull everything together and incorporate it into a plan in the following manner.

1) If you fail to plan you are planning to fail, so create a plan to adopt the program in "manageable bites" into your life.

2) As you are incorporating the program, refer to this section as needed for a quick review of any of the key points. If something doesn't make sense, go back and read the chapter in this book providing full detail on the key point.

3) Continue to expand your knowledge in the area of health. One of the most efficient ways to do this is to read my free twice-weekly e-newsletter, search for further detail on any topic at Mercola.com, and delve into the other resources covered in the Appendix.

A Simple Plan To Incorporate The Program Into Your Life

1) Use the test in Chapter 5 to get a basic idea of your metabolic type, or use the advanced online test described in that chapter to get a finer sense of your type. Start by eating in the general range of the macronutrient proportions for your type and, most importantly, begin the process of listening to your body and fine-tuning your macronutrients to your body's needs accordingly. The recipes in this book will help you toward that end.

2) At the beginning of your plan, anticipate if there are any emotional barriers, as discussed in Chapter 6, that will challenge your ability to implement this program. Do you already hear yourself saying something like, "There is no way I can give up sweets?" Have you encountered emotional barriers when trying to implement a healthy diet before? If you do anticipate any such barriers, incorporate the extremely effective Emotional Freedom Technique (defined in Chapter 6), or some other emotional/mental healing methodology, right at the outset. If and when you encounter any emotional barriers at any phase of implementing this program, pull out the "big guns" of EFT or some other approach as soon as possible so you don't abandon the program and your health, altogether. If you are not able

to obtain the results you are seeking with EFT, I would strongly advise you to seek one of the many well-trained EFT professionals that are out there to help guide you in this process.

3) As you're fine-tuning the proportions of macronutrients that are right for your type, you should also be abandoning the forms of those macronutrients that are unhealthy and adopting the forms that are healthy. I'd recommend cutting added sugars and processed grains, and cutting unhealthy meats and fish and replacing with healthy ones, first and fore-most. You should establish a timeline for yourself and a list of small steps to reach your bigger goals.

4) You should also begin incorporating the lifestyle changes covered in the previous chapter and summarized below into your life. I recommend drinking clean water and taking essential supplements such as fish oil should be among your very first priorities.

5) You should create a timeline with specific goals set in each period of time to work toward, all the way through complete adoption of this program. This is the ideal plan to integrate the program in stages.

A Sample Plan

It is well established that the very act of writing goals greatly increases your likelihood of achieving them. Unfortunately less than 3% of people write out their goals. I can tell you person-ally that writing out my goals has been one of the most profoundly beneficial things I have done. Once you have your goals, you will need to implement them, so I would also highly recommend that you purchase a copy of the book Getting Things Done by David Allen. It is an incredible collection of practical details that will help you clear up any "clutter" in your life so you will have more room to implement the changes that are discussed in this book. You can order this book at a discount through Mercola.com.

Below is an example of how you can establish a plan for yourself. I highly recommend you write your plan out and place it somewhere where you'll be reminded of it daily to help you stay on track.

In this case, the plan is laid out on a monthly basis that seems to work well for many people, but of course you can establish any increments of time that work for you. You should also consider planning for the next three to six months at most, after which point you should create a new plan incorporating new goals and any previous goals you didn't achieve to your satisfaction.

While I do recommend the goals laid out in the first month below be among your first priorities as well, you know best what health concerns you have for yourself and therefore what goals you first want to achieve, so plan for yourself accordingly. You can use the key points in the next section to help you plan, and of course if there are other health goals you have that aren't covered here, you can work those into your plan as well.

The amount of goals in each month below may seem just right, too minimal, or too aggressive for you; only you know what "manageable bites" means to you, so plan accordingly. If after awhile you find that you've bitten off more than you can chew, or achieving your goals is too easy, you can adjust it accordingly. And finally, you'll notice that the top goal in every month after the first is to work on completing any goals from previous months that have not been achieved to your satisfaction. It is important to include this in your plan, as it is a reminder that you're only human, and it is only counterproductive to get frustrated or give up if you're not being superhuman—success doesn't mean you'll achieve all of the goals all of the time on the first (or second or third) go-around, but instead that you'll keep trying to do so. To keep trying to improve, after all, is how optimal health is achieved.

Month One
- After learning my metabolic type, start fine-tuning to determine my ideal level of macronutrients
- Start using Emotional Freedom Technique to address what I feel is an addiction to sweets
- Start cutting the added sugars and processed grains from my diet
- Start eating more of the right vegetables for my carbohydrate needs
- Use only healthy, naturally raised meats in my meals
- Start taking fish oil, vitamin E, and probiotics daily, eliminate the unnecessary supplements I am taking
- Drink only clean water; have my tap water tested and appropriate filter installed

Month Two
- Keep working toward any of the goals from the previous month that are not at the level I want them to be yet
- Get eight hours of sleep per night, and try to go to bed and awake at same time daily
- Start exercising by walking for thirty minutes per day
- Stop drinking pasteurized milk, start eating grass-fed organic cheese and try to find source for raw milk

Month Three
- Keep working toward any of the goals from previous two months that are not at the level I want them to be yet
- Cut whole grains from my diet
- Start using only coconut oil and olive oil in my recipes
- Start trying to buy organic produce as much as I can
- Increase my exercise to 45 minutes per day

Month Four
- Keep working toward any of the goals from previous three months that are not at the level I want them to be yet
- Increase exercise to sixty minutes per day and incorporate weight training
- Start learning a meditation technique or some technique to manage my stress

Key Points of Dr. Mercola's Total Health Program

You can use these key points of my dietary and lifestyle program as reminders of all you have read, and to establish your personal plan.

Eating Healthy Foods

- Eliminate or vastly reduce grains from your diet.
- Eliminate sugar from your diet.
- Most of your daily carbohydrates should come from vegetables.
- Eat organically grown vegetables and fruits.
- Eat beans and legumes in moderation.
- Avoid soybeans and most soy products.
- Nuts and seeds are good in moderation.
- Fish, cod liver, coconut, and olive oil are very nutritious oils.
- Make sure you include traditionally fermented foods like healthy kefir in your diet.
- Grass-fed beef, bison, ostrich, and limited quantities of lamb, and free-ranged and organic chicken, turkey and other poultry are excellent protein sources.
- Avoid fish that hasn't been laboratory tested and shown to be free of mercury and other toxins.
- Organic, free-ranged eggs eaten raw are an excellent source of protein.
- Drinking raw milk and eating raw grass-fed cheese are excellent dairy choices.

Fine-Tuning for Your Metabolic Type

- Learn your metabolic type and follow the recommendations for your type.
- Learn to listen to your body and fine-tune your diet to reach the ideal level of macronutrients for you.

Addressing Your Emotional Health

- Determine what your emotional barriers to dietary and health success are.
- Learn EFT or obtain professional EFT or energy psychology assistance.
- Discover the benefits of prayer or meditation, and remember to take time to enjoy life.

Other Essential Steps to Optimal Health

- Drink at least eight glasses of clean water per day.
- Make exercise a routine part of your life.
- Get at least 7 to 9 hours of sleep per night.
- Supplement your diet with fish or cod liver oil, vitamin E, probiotics, and chlorella.
- Try Living Fuel for a quick and healthy meal replacement.

9: Take Control of Your Health for Good By Staying Informed

The foundation of my entire program, as you certainly understand by now, is that you need to take charge of your own health. The conventional healthcare system is controlled by drug companies that have profit and power far ahead of you on their agendas.

The single most important step you can take to stay in charge of your health is to remain informed. The program described in Part One of this book provides a rock-solid foundation to build your health upon. But health is an ever-evolving field, so you should strive to remain aware of the important findings that can help you. I urge you to subscribe to my free health e-newsletter at Mercola.com, to access the 30,000 pages of information at Mercola.com whenever you need insight on a specific health topic, and to take advantage of the other health resources in the Appendix.

If you aren't already a subscriber you should definitely consider my free e-newsletter and Mercola.com to keep informed of all the breaking health news that can make a major difference in your life. What you'll get—on a twice-weekly basis with my free e-newsletter, on a daily basis with my "Health Blog" link on Mercola.com—is the most important and up-to-date information that you can personally use in fighting and preventing specific diseases and common illnesses, managing weight, improving mental and emotional health, and generally feeling better and living longer. You'll find food and health product reviews and recommendations unbiased by outside influences, as Mercola.com is not tied in with any third parties or "sponsors" and accepts no form of advertising dollars. And you'll also receive my insight and the insight of other experts on our current healthcare fiasco and what to do about it. Mercola.com is not tied into—and therefore not constrained or manipulated by—any third party, and my only policy is to provide you the truth, backed by years of my own and other contributors' expertise, of what can really help you.

For your sake, take action with this dietary and lifestyle program. Many people read "how-to" information, but unfortunately never actually use it, but you can do this program, you will succeed with it, and I've seen it thousands of times—you will love yourself for doing it. Enjoy the delicious and nutritious recipes in Part Two, continue to expand your knowledge base, believe in yourself, and welcome to an incredible health transformation!

PART TWO
THE RECIPES

10: Equipping Your Kitchen, and Yourself, for Healthy Cooking

Congratulations! You've read through Part One of this book and are now fully equipped with the right knowledge for your journey to optimal health. You are just about ready to start using the recipes here in Part Two, but before you begin, there are just a couple more things you should know to use them most effectively: how to prepare your kitchen for the healthiest and most time-efficient food preparation, and how these recipes are arranged to help you follow your metabolic type.

Equipping Your Kitchen

For starters, the type of cookware and utensils you use can definitely impact the nutritional value of food. It is, first of all, important to use cookware with non-reactive surfaces. Aluminum and "non-stick" cookware are both highly toxic, and should not be used. Aluminum, also found in baking powder, anti-acids, antiperspirants, unfiltered tap water and even table salt, is a very soft, reactive metal that is easily absorbed by the body. It can be dangerous, even fatal, if consumed in excessive amounts, and has been implicated in the development of many diseases including Alzheimer's. The chemical reaction of high-acid foods like tomatoes with aluminum causes the metal to leach or migrate into the food. So, foods like spaghetti sauce made in an aluminum pot are a disaster waiting to happen.

Synthetic, non-stick coatings are no better. They're easily scratched with regular metal utensils, enabling flecks of the coating to get into your food. In two to five minutes on a conventional stovetop, cookware coated with Teflon and other non-stick surfaces can also reach excessive temperatures at which the coating breaks apart and emits toxic particles and gases, including carcinogens, global pollutants, and MFA, a chemical lethal to humans at low doses. Is the so-called convenience of these non-stick coatings really worth these risks? Professional chefs and restaurateurs use stainless steel equipment and you should also. Spun-steel woks, glass and ironclad porcelain cookware are also safe cookware to use.

The microwave oven is another piece of "convenience" equipment you are strongly encouraged to avoid. Microwave ovens cause destructive chemical and structural changes to food. This includes formation of unnatural radiolytic compounds that can negatively impact your health.

Here are a few key insights to consider about certain tools and appliances that are ideal for your kitchen:

Knives

The most indispensable of the kitchen tools, knives are often the most neglected. For best life and performance, and to prevent accidents, make sure your knives are kept sharp with a butcher's steel or knife sharpener. There is a knife for every job. A set of six quality, precision hard steel knives, properly cared for, can last a lifetime. Proper care means frequent sharpening, drying immediately after use, and storing in a knife rack or on a magnetic bar, not jumbled carelessly with other kitchen tools in a kitchen drawer.

Electric Blender and Food Processors

These are both needed and are the most useful appliances in the kitchen. You will use them frequently for chopping nuts and vegetables, and blending shakes, soups, and sauces. It is not necessary to get a high priced model, just a highly rated model. For example, when my $400 Vitamixer broke, I went to Amazon.com to look at the user ratings for blenders and found a highly rated Black and Decker blender for $25. I love it and would never spend $400 on a blender again.

Juicer

One of the most convenient and delicious ways to get the maximum quantity and quality of nutrient-rich vegetables and fruits is the vegetable juice extractor. You can use it to make fresh juices, smoothies, soups and stocks in virtually seconds. Circulating blades extract or "squeeze" out the valuable juice, leaving only the pulpy fiber, which can also be used to add bulk to healthy snacks, confections and other recipes. In addition to juicing, many juicers can also chop and grind food, so they are a great value. Hands down, the best juicer on the market is the Omega 8002 Juicer. See the extensive juicer comparison table evaluating a range of brands and their features in the Recommended Products section on Mercola.com, where the Omega 8002 came out a clear winner in terms of ease of use and cleaning, durability, versatility and price.

Wok

One of the oldest and still one of the most useful of all cooking utensils is the wok, a large, heavy, round-bottomed pan with a cover, used by the Chinese for centuries. The food cooks efficiently because the wok sits on a ring over the burner, concentrating the heat. With it you can efficiently and quickly sauté, stew, deep-fry, steam or get a meal on the table in only a few minutes using the famous "stir-fry" technique. A flat skillet can be used for stir-frying, but the wok's round bottom and ring fit over the burner perfectly, concentrating the heat and allowing you to sauté foods in stages, cooking everything in one pan. Purchase a cold spun-steel wok, at least 12" in diameter, from an Asian cooking specialty store or restaurant supply house. Don't even bother with the cheaper aluminum, electrically-fired wok imposters.

Crockpot

Another inexpensive but truly timesaving kitchen appliance is the crockpot, which many people come to appreciate especially during colder weather. This freestanding electrical appliance can be invaluable for preparing soups, stews, casseroles and other winter meals, especially if you are work-ing full-time outside the home. The preferred cooking insert is ceramic, which can be filled with the makings for a one-dish meat and vegetable casserole or a stew that can simmer at a very low temperature while you are away during the day, yielding a fully prepared meal, ready when you walk in the door.

Dehydrator

Drying is one of the oldest ways to preserve food. A food dehydrator is a low cost, low-fuss way to process and preserve fresh vegetables and other foods that can then be stored at room temperature. A dehydrator works by removing excess water from food by continuously circulating thermostatically controlled, low heat air over the food in the chamber. The thermostat range is usually between 85°F and 145°F. Below 115°F–118°F, the food is not cooked, so you can prepare vegetable-based crackers, sandwich wraps, fruit and veggie "leathers" that are healthy and technically still raw. The dehydrator is an ideal and economical way to process large quantities of fresh, local, organic or biodynamically grown fruits and vegetables you might acquire in season. There are many available on the market, but the Excalibur is one of the best brands.

Seed or Coffee Grinder

A coffee grinder is excellent for grinding small quantities of nuts, seeds, spices and other hard foods. It is especially good for flax seeds, which should always been ground right before using.

Spiral Slicer

The Spiral Slicer™ is a versatile, manual tool that performs a number of vegetable processing tasks, including making various cuts, slices, half slices, strips, strands and decorative spirals. Its best feature is its ability to make long, thin, continuous strands of vegetables like zucchini and kohlrabi, turning them into authentic-looking pasta, a great treat for people following my grain-free dietary program.

Safe Food Storage and Handling

As detailed throughout my Total Health Program, the fresher and more natural your foods, whether plant- or animal-based, the better they are for you. Storing these foods, though, is also critical to maintain their health, and your own. Old, spoiled or devitalized food is a waste of money that can also be a health hazard. Leftovers or food that is being prepared for future use should always be cooled down as rapidly as possible and stored in containers with a cover in the refriger-ator. Do not hold or use leftover cooked food for more than three days. Even if it hasn't gone bad, it will certainly be devitalized.

When grocery shopping, place the produce in a plastic bag and push all the air out of the bag before sealing it with a twist tie, as this will keep the produce fresh longer. Upon returning from a shopping trip, make sure to get your produce and other foods into the refrigerator, freezer or cold storage area as soon as possible. Moist foods like lettuce and fresh herbs should be washed, drained, sorted, and bagged before refrigerating, but do not wash mushrooms until you are ready to use them. Dry foods like onions and winter squashes should not be refrigerated, but kept at lower room temperature. Don't remove food from the refrigerator until just before you are ready to use it, and return immediately after use. When thawing foods, do so in the refrigerator or in cold water in your sink, never at room temperature.

The best food storage containers are non-reactive, reusable ones, especially glass and ceramic containers with tight-fitting lids. You can obtain reusable vacuum seal stoppers for removing the oxygen from already opened bottles, which are very helpful for preventing oxidation and preserving the quality of raw oils and freshly prepared juices. Plastic is ubiquitous these days as a food packaging and storage material, but is the least desirable storage material because it can leach into your food. Try using more of the renewable materials for your food carting and storage, such as wax paper, butcher and brown paper, glass, ceramic, enamel, wood and cloth, as they are healthier for you (and the planet) than plastic. I personally put all my leftovers in bell jars and I seal them with a canning device called the FoodSaver Vac 1050 (go to www.tilia.com) to remove the oxygen that causes the food to oxidize (spoil).

Organizing Yourself

The key to reducing the time you spend preparing your meals is to invest more time up front in planning. By taking the following steps, you will not only greatly reduce the amount of time you spend in the kitchen, but you will also avoid the temptation of last-minute conveniences that often leads to health problems.

- Plan your meals in advance
- Organize your food stock
- Shop intentionally, based on what you need
- Prepare your meals at a set time and prepare them efficiently

Plan Your Meals, Your Food Stock, and Your Shopping

Once a week, set aside some time to plan your meals for the upcoming week. You can do this with pen and paper, or there are recipe planning calendars that you can find at most bookstores or more sophisticated diet and recipe planning software such as Diet Pro and Living Cookbook you can find online at radiumtechnologies.com.

If the habit of planning your meals in advance is new to you, the recipes in this book are a great place to start. Leaf through the pages and find all the recipes that appeal to you, and that are a good starting point for fine-tuning your diet to your metabolic type. Schedule the recipes you want to try on specific days throughout the week. Ideally this would include breakfast, lunch, and dinner, as the more meals you can schedule, the more successful you'll generally be. Be sure to stay realistic about your life and work schedule and plan appropriately. Regarding snacks, you should even pencil in what snacks you'll want to make and have on hand for that week.

By planning out your meals in this manner, you will spare yourself the daily stress of not knowing what to eat or how long it will take you to prepare it, and from caving in to eating unhealthy fast or prepackaged foods. If you are traveling, you'll also want to plan accordingly, perhaps including a healthy convenience food like Living Fuel (see Chapter 7 or Recommended Ingredients and Product Locator in the Appendix) in your plan, or at least proactively planning what type of food you will eat at a restaurant.

When you plan your shopping list each week in this manner, you'll also be able to plan what foods you need to stock and therefore shop for only the foods you need. This intentional shopping will save multiple trips to the store and help you avoid impulse purchases of junk food.

Schedule Time For Efficient Meal Preparation

It is highly beneficial to schedule your food preparation at the same time on a routine basis. This helps it quickly become a habit you don't even have to think about, like going to bed and waking up at the same time every day.

"Batch cooking" is one of the most efficient ways to prepare healthy meals and save yourself time, especially if you are cooking for a family. This is the method of cooking several days' worth of meals at one time versus having to cook every day. For instance, you can roast a chicken or turkey for a Sunday dinner that will yield valuable protein for main dishes and lunches during the week. You could prepare two oven casseroles while the bird is roasting. After dinner, you could bone, cut up and bag some of the leftover chicken for Roll-Ups or chicken salad, and simmer the bones to create a homemade stock that could easily become soup.

The key is to regularly schedule one long or two shorter blocks of time for these batch cooking sessions where you are preparing enough for several days worth of eating. It allows you to efficiently produce a variety of completed or partially completed meals that can be: 1) eaten fresh; 2) stored properly as previously discussed and consumed within the next two days; and/or 3) placed in the freezer to be pulled out as needed for quick suppers and lunches during the week.

11: How These Recipes are Arranged

The recipes that Nancy Lee Bentley has created are a unique mix of classic and traditional, American and international fare, with both healthy gourmet and down-home influences. In the recipes you will also find a multi-dimensional mix of ingredients, techniques and principles taken from a very wide range of cooking and food preparation philosophies and schools. Many are actually adapted from French and other classical cooking techniques, and also borrow from Italian, Greek, Brazilian, African, German and other international cuisines.

But for all the nuances that make each of them distinct and delicious, they still all have one thing in common—they're geared to help you adopt and master my dietary program and eat according to your metabolic type. While these recipes are designed for ease-of-preparation and delicious taste, they're also centered on using the healthiest forms of foods that, as you know by now, are essential to preventing disease, optimizing weight, increasing energy and a youthful appearance, and prolonging your life. And they're designed to help you learn. The main recipe on each page is always the one best suited for a Mixed Metabolic Type, but as appropriate for each recipe, the guidelines for Protein and Carb Types to properly prepare the recipe are included. Tips and notes accompany each recipe to provide further insight to all metabolic types on how to fine-tune the recipe, or add other recipes, to make it most suitable for their nutritional needs.

In a short time, by working with these recipes and following the advice in each of them, you will become an expert at "listening to your body" and fine-tuning these recipes and recipes from any source to your particular health needs.

The following is important information for understanding the cookbook:

- The main recipe that appears on the page is always a Mixed Type or "MX" recipe.

- Protein Types (PT) and Carb Types (CT) need to look under "Cooking Tips" on each recipe page for specific instructions for varying the recipe to fit Protein and Carb Types.

- Many main recipes contain no meat or can be prepared without adding animal protein. You will also find some "No-Meat Mains" geared to vegetarians in the Main Dishes chapter.

- All of the recipes have been developed with busy people in mind. The recipes average 15 minutes preparation time or less.

- If you can't find a particular food, check the Appendix of this book for recommendations on how to obtain it.

How the Recipes are Organized on the Page

The following recipes are logically organized according to each major type of dish or food group, such as Main Dishes, Desserts, etc. Each of these sections begins with an introduction that provides some specific information about the foods and recipes that follow.

Note that all the recipes use the following abbreviations:

MX   =   Mixed Type
PT   =   Protein Type
CT   =   Carbohydrate Type

Many of these recipes are actually three recipes in one. The main recipe you see on the page is always the Mixed Type (MX) recipe. If you have determined that you're a Protein or Carb Type, though, you'll find specific instructions for adjusting and varying the recipes to your needs in the "Cooking Tips" area of each recipe.

To help you learn and perfect this fine-tuning and eating properly for your metabolic type, the "Notes and Suggestions" section of each recipe contains 1) ideas for creating metabolically balanced meals and menus; 2) suggestions to help you listen to your body, monitor your reactions, and work on fine-tuning the proportions for your specific type.

Customizing These Recipes to YOUR Total Health

As you understand by now, these recipes provide far more than just a list of ingredients and the procedures for putting them together. They are actually tools—tools that taste great—for incorporating my entire dietary program into your life so you can prevent disease, optimize your weight permanently, and live longer. They put the lessons from Part One about the right types of foods into play, and they teach you how to vary and customize your food intake for your specific metabolic needs. Remember these general macronutrient ratios for each metabolic type back in Chapter 5:

General Macronutrient Ratios

Mixed Type: 30% Proteins / 20% Fats / 50% Carbohydrates
Protein Type: 40% Proteins / 30% Fats / 30% Carbohydrates
Carb Type: 25% Proteins / 15% Fats / 60% Carbohydrates

These are starting benchmarks for the amount of macronutrients you should generally try to consume daily, but instead of getting hung up on these numbers, it is much more important to listen to your body—your own natural feedback mechanism that will tell you if what you consume is right or not—to determine your ideal macronutrient ratios.

This whole process of fine-tuning is about becoming more aware of what your body is telling you. You've got an excellent starting point by knowing your basic metabolic type, and by understanding what foods you should be eating and avoiding, so now—because only you are in control of your own body—the rest is up to you. Since your goal is total health, do not be afraid to experiment with these recipes, or any aspect of your daily food intake. Adjust the levels and even types of ingredients and assess how you feel up to two hours later—when you feel great as discussed in Chapter 5, you are doing something quite right for your body. Throw out the "rules" about eating certain kinds of foods at breakfast versus lunch and dinner and instead adopt the recipes that make you feel best for any meal of the day. Who said you can't eat soup in the morning anyway? That said, enjoy!

THE RECIPES: Salads

Salads are most people's first encounter with raw foods. Quick and easy to make, they are an easy and delicious way to consume 30–50% of your daily food in a raw state.

Remember that organic vegetables are generally both healthier and tastier. The best way to begin this program is to focus on the vegetables recommended for your metabolic type; consult the Recommended Foods Tables in Chapter 5 as needed. Carefully monitor how you feel after eating these vegetables, and continue to monitor as you expand into trying other vegetables. You'll find these salad recipes are a delicious way to experiment with nature's healthiest foods, and to help you fine-tune your diet.

You can choose to keep wishing you were thinner, healthier, and younger looking but not take the steps to actually improve your health. Or you can choose to make achieving optimal health a true priority in your life, and dedicate yourself to achieving it through the proven advice, recipes, and resources this book offers. Read on if your health and life are worth that effort.

Aegean Salad

An authentic Greek salad, especially good with summer's fresh garden bounty.

2¹/₂	med cucumber, peeled, seeded and diced
1	med tomato, seeded and chopped
¹/₃	cup green pepper, minced
8	pitted black olives, cut into quarters
1	med scallion, sliced
3	Tbsp feta cheese
¹/₄	cup red wine vinegar
2¹/₂	Tbsp extra virgin olive oil
1	Tbsp fresh oregano, chopped, or 1 tsp dried
	salt and pepper to taste

Nutrition Facts

	calories	total fat	carbs	protein
Mixed Type:	145	12g	8g	3g
Carb Type:	100	7g	9g	3g
Protein Type:	173	14g	10g	5g

Cooking Tips

PT: Not really a PT kind of salad, but adding 2 cups tiny cauliflowerettes and reducing cucumbers to 2, using 4 chopped anchovy filets and increasing olives to 3 Tbsp could help. Use 2 Tbsp extra virgin olive oil.

CT: Add 1 cucumber. Reduce feta cheese to 2 Tbsp and olive oil to 1 Tbsp. Decrease black olives to 2 per person, quartered.

Notes and Suggestions

For a complete Greek meal, combine this salad with the Greek Egg-Lemon Soup and Basic Roast Chicken. Opa!

1 combine diced cucumber, chopped tomato, green pepper, black olives and sliced scallion in large mixing or serving bowl.

2 crumble feta cheese over top. Drizzle vinegar and olive oil over salad. Sprinkle with salt, pepper and oregano. Toss at the table just before serving.

Serves 4. Preparation time: 5 minutes.

Chop Chop Garden Salad

A rainbow of garden colors, flavors and crunchy goodness.

2	cups broccoli flowerettes
1	cup cauliflowerettes
¾	cup chopped parsley
2	sprigs fresh marjoram or 1½ tsp dried
1	med shallot, finely chopped
1	8-oz pkg clover sprouts
6	radishes, chopped
2	Tbsp Basic Sunny Seed Mix (page 219)
2	Tbsp extra virgin olive oil
2	grinds fresh black pepper
3	spritz Bragg's Liquid Aminos (about ½ tsp)

1 chop broccoli and cauliflower until coarsely chopped.

2 combine with parsley, marjoram, shallot, sprouts, radishes, and seed mix in a large serving bowl.

3 drizzle with oil, sprinkle with pepper, and spritz with Bragg's. Toss and serve.

Serves 4. Preparation time: 10 minutes.

Nutrition Facts

	calories	total fat	carbs	protein
Mixed Type:	89	7g	6g	3g
Carb Type:	75	5g	7g	3g
Protein Type:	118	10g	6g	3g

Cooking Tips

PT: Use 3 cups cauliflower and 1 cup broccoli flowerettes. Increase seed mix to 4 Tbsp.

CT: Add 1 cup peeled and diced broccoli stems and increase parsley to 1½ cups. Reduce oil to 1⅓ Tbsp and seed mix to 1 Tbsp.

Notes and Suggestions

A crunchy, colorful vegetable salad, ideal for CT, this variation on the Southern favorite "chop" salad can be served as a side dish with just about any meat entrée. Or combine it with a soup like Blended Broccoli, Asparagus and Artichoke, or Creamy Avocado, and add additional protein, such as turkey bacon, cooked leftover turkey for PT, fresh mozzarella, lowfat farmer or cottage cheese, if you are a CT.

Creamy Eggplant Tossed Salad

This quick, yet creamy, smooth dressing adds a perfect contrast to the broiled eggplant and leafy greens.

½	lb med eggplant
1	tsp sea salt
½	tsp poultry seasoning or thyme leaves
½	tsp dried basil or oregano
1	large head leaf lettuce
1	med cucumber, shredded & patted dry
½	cup cooked turkey cubes
2	tsp capers, drained
¼	cup Sunny Seed Salad Dressing (page 237)

Nutrition Facts

	calories	total fat	carbs	protein
Mixed Type:	209	10g	18g	18g
Carb Type:	134	4g	13g	13g
Protein Type:	279	15g	18g	221g

Cooking Tips

PT: Substitute fresh baby spinach for most of the lettuce, adding 2 cups torn leaf lettuce. Increase dark meat turkey to ³⁄4 cup and salad dressing to ¹⁄3 cup.

CT: Increase cucumber to 2, reduce salad dressing to 1 Tbsp.

Notes and Suggestions

This is a quick and delicious mini-meal salad with unique flavors and textures. This can become a main meal salad by adding more of the appropriate type of light or dark, cooked poultry meat, so it is a fast way to fix lunch when you have leftover roast turkey or chicken (or even pheasant) after the weekend.

1 turn on broiler. Cut eggplant into ¼" slices. Place eggplant slices on cookie sheet. Sprinkle with salt, poultry seasoning, and basil.

2 broil approximately 3–4 minutes per side, until eggplant slices start to brown. Remove from heat.

3 meanwhile, tear washed lettuce into large serving bowl. Add cucumber to salad along with turkey cubes. Cut up broiled eggplant into chunks and add to salad with capers.

4 pour dressing over salad and toss.

Serves 2. Preparation time: 15 minutes.

Fresh Mozzarella Plate

The Italians' favorite Calabrese salad makes use of fresh tomatoes, basil, and mozzarella cheese. Simple, spectacular, delicious!

2	med cucumbers, peeled and thinly sliced
½	lb fresh mozzarella cheese, sliced
1	cup cherry tomatoes, halved
1	cup fresh basil leaves, packed
1	tsp sea or celtic salt
10	grinds fresh black pepper
2	Tbsp extra virgin olive oil

1 assemble serving plates. Layer overlapping slices of cucumber on plates. Top with fresh mozzarella slices.

2 arrange cherry tomato pieces and sprigs of fresh basil on cheese.

3 sprinkle with sea salt and pepper. Drizzle delicately with olive oil. Serve.

Serves 4. Preparation time: 5 minutes.

Nutrition Facts

	calories	total fat	carbs	protein
Mixed Type:	260	20g	7g	14g
Carb Type:	211	13g	9g	16g
Protein Type:	260	20g	7g	16g

Cooking Tips

PT: Use whole milk, fresh mozzarella cheese, the small round white balls in tubs of water, usually found in deli or better cheese section. Try using 3 cups fresh, cooled, steamed asparagus instead of cucumber.

CT: Use lowfat mozzarella. Increase cucumbers to 3. You might want to add a small jar of drained, roasted red peppers to this antipasto-type plate.

Notes and Suggestions

This favorite summer salad plate could become a full antipasto meal spread with the addition of sliced buffalo summer sausage, sardines, pepperoncini peppers, marinated mushrooms or black olives. Probably would appeal more to a PT or MX type.

Frilly French Brunch Salad

This adaptation of a light French Bistro Salad, reminiscent of Eggs Benedict, is ideal for a Sunday brunch or any lunch.

2	heads frisée or curly endive lettuce
4	slices turkey bacon, cut into small pieces
1	med scallion or green onion, sliced
1	Tbsp extra virgin olive oil
2	Tbsp apple cider vinegar
2	tsp Dijon mustard
¼	tsp sea salt
3	grinds black pepper
6	eggs

Nutrition Facts

	calories	total fat	carbs	protein
Mixed Type:	192	14g	4g	13g
Carb Type:	156	11g	4g	10g
Protein Type:	243	16g	6g	20g

Cooking Tips

PT: Could substitute spinach for half of the greens. Use 8 slices of turkey bacon and 8 eggs. How about spooning warm Hollandaise sauce (page 176), 1 Tbsp per person, over the gently cooked egg, instead of drizzling salad with vinaigrette?

CT: Might find it more appealing to use lemon juice instead of vinegar. Use only 4 eggs in this recipe.

Notes and Suggestions

This is a standalone main dish salad that could be served at almost any meal. PT's should monitor level of satiety or satisfaction and increase protein, if still hungry after eating.

1 wash, drain and tear lettuce. Place in large serving bowl.

2 sauté turkey bacon in skillet over medium until crisp. Remove and sprinkle over greens.

3 add sliced scallion to skillet and sauté 1 minute. Remove from heat.

4 whisk olive oil, vinegar, mustard, salt and pepper to blend. Pour over greens. Toss.

5 heat two fingers of water to boiling in medium pan. Add a dash of vinegar and reduce to medium low. Break eggs, one at a time into small cup, then carefully slip eggs into simmering water. Poach 3–4 minutes only.

6 divide salad onto individual serving plates. Remove lightly poached eggs with slotted spoon and place atop each serving. Serve immediately.

Serves 4. Preparation time: 15 minutes.

Greek Cucumbers

A traditional cucumbers and cream side dish as an accompaniment to a lamb, fish or meat entrée.

3	med cucumbers
1/2	tsp sea salt
1/2	tsp celery seed
1/4	cup sour cream
1/2	cup plain yogurt
1	tsp red wine vinegar
2	cloves garlic, minced
	parsley flakes or dill weed

1 peel, seed and slice cucumbers into wing cuts in serving bowl.*

2 add salt, celery seed, sour cream, yogurt, vinegar, and minced garlic. Mix well. Garnish, sprinkled with parsley flakes or dill weed. Serve immediately.

Serves 2. Preparation time: 10 minutes.

Nutrition Facts

	calories	total fat	carbs	protein
Mixed Type:	143	5g	16g	6g
Carb Type:	68	1g	10g	4g
Protein Type:	164	6g	23g	9g

Cooking Tips

PT: Not really a PT salad, unless you want to exchange 3 cups of cauliflowerettes for cucumbers, use 1/2 cup sour cream, and 1/4 cup plain yogurt. Serve 3.

CT: Just your kind of salad, but add another cucumber and substitute 3/4 cup lowfat yogurt for the dairy.

*You can create wing cuts by cutting a peeled cucumber in half lengthwise, scooping out the seeds and slicing halves crosswise.

Notes and Suggestions

This side salad is a nice contrast to a plain meat entrée such as Grilled Lemon Salmon, Turkey Cutlets, Roast Chicken, or a plain Broiled Steak for a PT or MX. Add another vegetable dish such as Grecian Spinach or Braised Brazilian Greens for a balanced meal.

Grilled Ratatouille Salad

A jiffy version of the classical summer Ratatouille Provencal, presented this time as a salad that can be broiled indoors or grilled alongside chicken or beef in the backyard.

¼	cup extra virgin olive oil
½	lb eggplant, cut into ½" slices
¼	lb zucchini squash, cut into ½" slices
¼	lb yellow squash, cut in quarters
1	med red pepper, seeded and cut into quarters
1	small red onion, trimmed, cut into rings
¼	lb Roma or plum tomatoes, halved
4	med Portabella mushrooms, cut into halves
4	whole garlic cloves
1	4 oz can black olives, drained
	Tbsp dried oregano

Nutrition Facts

	calories	total fat	carbs	protein
Mixed Type:	256	17g	24g	7g
Carb Type:	204	11g	26g	7g
Protein Type:	295	22g	24g	7g

Cooking Tips

PT: Double the amount of mushrooms and decrease eggplant to 4 slices.

CT: Decrease olive oil to 2 Tbsp. Use a sprayer or pastry brush to lightly coat vegetables with oil. Skip all but 2 black olives per serving.

Notes and Suggestions

In addition to being a perfect partner for a barbecue, this delicious grilled vegetable dish could easily become a whole antipasto-type meal salad, with the addition of protein such as organic buffalo or beef summer sausage for PT, leftover grilled or BBQ chicken breast for CT.

1 brush eggplant, zucchini, yellow squash, peppers, onion rings, tomatoes, and mushrooms with olive oil.

2 grill vegetables over gas grill, charcoal, or even under your oven broiler, 3–5 minutes on a side, until translucent and partially blackened. Cool slightly. Cut into large chunks and arrange on large platter or shallow serving bowl.

3 cut garlic and olives lengthwise into slices and then slivers. Mix with oregano leaves and sprinkle over arranged salad. Serve slightly warm or at room temperature.

Serves 4. Preparation time: 20 minutes.

Hot Asian Shiitake Slaw

This warming, spicy hot Asian-style coleslaw transforms those good-for-you green leafies into a delicious mushroom-enhanced salad.

2	Tbsp tamari soy sauce
2	Tbsp lemon juice
2	cloves garlic, minced
1	tsp wasabi powder or grated horseradish
1	Tbsp freshly grated ginger root
3	cups Napa cabbage
2	cups bok choy
1	Tbsp sesame oil
1	tsp roasted sesame oil
1½	cups shiitake or button mushrooms, sliced

1 wash and cut up the bok choy and Napa cabbage. Place in large serving bowl.

2 blend soy sauce, lemon juice, minced garlic, wasabi powder or grated horseradish, and grated ginger in medium-sized bowl, and then bring this marinade to a boil on oven.

3 heat a medium skillet or wok over medium high heat. Add sesame oils and then mushroom slices and cook mushroom slices until lightly browned.

4 spoon the mushrooms over the greens. Pour the boiling marinade over the mushrooms and greens. Toss gently to coat. Serve immediately.

Serves 4. Preparation time: 15 minutes.

Nutrition Facts

	calories	*total fat*	*carbs*	*protein*
Mixed Type:	128	4.5g	15g	6.5g
Carb Type:	99	3.5g	8g	6.5g
Protein Type:	161	4.5g	23g	7.5g

Cooking Tips

PT: Substitute half spinach for greens. Increase mushrooms to 3 cups.

CT: Reduce oil to 1 Tbsp total. Add at least 2 more cups of bok choy and/or Napa cabbage and omit or greatly reduce mushrooms.

Notes and Suggestions

PT's and MT's should monitor how you feel after eating this dish. You might want to add some sliced bison to the salad to add some protein. CT's may find this satisfying as-is or prefer to add additional greens.

K.I.S.S. Salad in a Flash

Probably the simplest salad you've seen, yet amazingly tasty, with so few ingredients and so little fuss.

1	cup finely chopped curly parsley
¾	cup shredded jicama
¼	cup finely shredded organic carrot
2	tsp extra virgin olive oil or grapeseed oil
1	Tbsp freshly squeezed lemon juice
¼	tsp Spike or Mrs. Dash vegetable seasoning

1 combine chopped parsley, shredded jicama and carrot.

2 sprinkle with olive oil, lemon juice, and vegetable seasoning. Toss and serve.

Serves 1. Preparation time: 5 minutes.

Nutrition Facts

	calories	total fat	carbs	protein
Mixed Type:	153	10g	16g	3g
Carb Type:	114	5g	16g	3g
Protein Type:	186	14g	15g	2g

Cooking Tips

PT: You can make this more for your type by substituting or adding spinach for part of the parsley. This will not have enough fat for you, so you will probably want to add at least 1 Tbsp of extra virgin olive oil.

CT: Use 1 tsp oil. This is your kind of dish, perfect as a salad accompaniment to soup or main entrée such as a stir-fry or stew.

Notes and Suggestions

Enjoy this fast and simple salad with some additional protein like salmon, eggs or low-fat cheese for a satisfying CT lunch. This is barely a snack for most PT's, but could be the salad accompaniment in a meat-based menu.

Kohlrabi and Side Kick Dippers

In the South they know it as "Garden Sass," a plate of just-picked garden fresh veggies. Pack or serve unusual vegetable sticks with a quick and easy "dry" dip for a doable lunch or snack on the go.

1	large or 3 med kohlrabi or turnips
4	med celery stalks
1	small jicama
1	red pepper, seeded
2	small yellow squash
2	cups broccoli flowerettes
1	cup snow pea pods
1/3	cup Sunny Seed Gomasio (page 215)

1 wash vegetables and pat dry. Peel, where appropriate and cut up into equal size sticks.

2 arrange on a large platter with a small bowl of Sunny Seed Gomasio topping in the center.

3 or divide up vegetables and serve a mixed selection of sticks with about 1 Tbsp Gomasio each (or more as desired).

4 serve, encouraging guests to roll or dip their veggie sticks into the dry topping. Unusual, but good!

Serves 4. Preparation time: 15 minutes.

Nutrition Facts

	calories	total fat	carbs	protein
Mixed Type:	140	4g	24g	6g
Carb Type:	98	1g	22g	4g
Protein Type:	176	6g	28g	8g

Cooking Tips

PT: Will need to add more protein such as leftover meat or cheese. Double the celery and add whole green beans to optimize this for your type.

CT: Once again, this is an ideal type of dish for you, although minimize the amount and frequency of the gomasio, ground seeds. The savory, lightly toasted flavor goes a long way, so you won't need much.

Notes and Suggestions

A great idea to take along with you for a handy snack. You might want to purchase one of those small, soft-sided lunch boxes for toting your food essentials wherever you go. A great habit to cultivate!

Marinated Italian Salad

This distinctively Italian salad with its red, green, white, and black colors is a popular summer favorite. Goes together super fast and looks great on a buffet table in a tall glass container.

1	cup cherry tomatoes, halved and seeded
1	med green pepper, seeded
8	oz provolone or mozzarella cheese
¼	cup black olives, drained
1	med cucumber, seeded
1	med red onion
2–3	sprigs fresh basil leaves, torn, or 2 tsp dried basil
¼	cup extra virgin olive oil
2	Tbsp red wine vinegar
½	tsp sea salt
3–4	grinds freshly ground black pepper

1 cut vegetables and cheese into equal size cuts, about ½" each.

2 in large mixing bowl, combine cherry tomatoes, green pepper, cheese cubes, black olives, cucumber, onion, and basil leaves.

3 quickly whisk olive oil, vinegar, salt and pepper together to blend.

4 pour over salad and toss lightly to coat. Serve immediately or cover and marinate 1–2 hours in refrigerator.

Serves 5. Preparation time: 10 minutes.

Nutrition Facts

	calories	total fat	carbs	protein
Mixed Type:	290	24g	7g	13g
Carb Type:	184	12g	10g	9g
Protein Type:	339	29g	9g	13g

Cooking Tips

PT: An ideal salad for your type, heavy on protein and fat. You could increase olives to ³/4 cup and olive oil to ¹/3 cup. Add 2 stalks celery cut into appropriate size chunks. Use 10 oz cheese.

CT: Too high in fat as is, you can decrease the olives to 8 or so, cut in half. Use only half the cheese and use lowfat mozzarella. Add another cucumber to your recipe and serve 4.

Notes and Suggestions

This hearty salad can be made into another Italian antipasto-type meal salad, plated on a large flat platter lined with lettuce leaves. PT's can add anchovies, herring, marinated mussels, or cubes or slices of bison summer sausage or turkey ham. CT's might want to add radishes, jicama, pickled or fresh okra or Brussels sprouts to this colorful array.

Middle Eastern Salad

This no-grain version of Taboulleh, a Mediterranean favorite, is packed with anti-oxidant vitamins A and C.

2	cups curly parsley, chopped
2	cups flat-leaf Italian parsley, chopped
2	med cucumbers, peeled, seeded, finely diced
³⁄₄	cup finely chopped tomatoes
³⁄₄	cup finely diced celery
1	cup chopped fresh mint leaves
1	Tbsp pine nuts
2	Tbsp fresh lemon juice
2	Tbsp extra virgin olive oil
1	tsp salt
3	grinds fresh black pepper

1 combine curly and flat-leaf parsleys, cucumber, tomatoes, celery, mint leaves, and pine nuts in medium salad bowl.

2 mix lemon juice, olive oil, salt and pepper in small cup and pour over salad. Toss well to mix.

3 transfer to serving bowl or divide into servings on lettuce-lined plates. Serve immediately.

Serves 4. Preparation time: 10 minutes.

Nutrition Facts

	calories	*total fat*	*carbs*	*protein*
Mixed Type:	160	12g	12g	4g
Carb Type:	141	7g	17g	5g
Protein Type:	196	17g	10g	4g

Cooking Tips

PT: Substitute 1 cup chopped spinach for 1 cup of the parsley. Reduce tomatoes to ¹⁄₂ cup. Increase oil to 3 Tbsp. Use ¹⁄₄ cup pine nuts.

CT: Ideal for your type. Add 1 med chopped cucumber. Reduce olive oil to 1¹⁄₃ Tbsp. Sprinkle top with a few pine nuts. Serves 3.

Notes and Suggestions

This is a great summer salad, ideal for CT. To make it a meal salad, CT could add (2–3 oz) of feta cheese and some chopped egg. PT and MX could add chopped bison or organic beef summer sausage, or serve with additional protein like marinated herring.

Northwoods Broccoli Salad

Reminiscent of that popular broccoli-bacon-raisin deli salad with an up North twist.

2	heads organic broccoli
1/2	small red onion, minced
2	Tbsp dried cranberries, minced
6	strips turkey bacon, chopped
1/2	cup mayonnaise
1/4	cup plain organic yogurt
1/4	cup organic walnuts, chopped

Nutrition Facts

	calories	total fat	carbs	protein
Mixed Type:	313	20g	31g	9g
Carb Type:	134	10g	9g	4g
Protein Type:	318	18g	32g	14g

Cooking Tips

PT: Use 1 head broccoli and 1 head cauliflower. Use 8 strips turkey bacon and increase walnuts to 1/3 cup. Substitute currants for dried cranberries.

CT: Reduce bacon to 2 strips. Use 1/4 cup mayo and 1/2 cup plain nonfat yogurt. Reduce walnuts to 2 Tbsp chopped, sprinkled on top.

Notes and Suggestions

This hearty, cold weather salad would be a nice accompaniment to a chili or stew, or another type of crockpot meal such as Crockpot Chicken Curry or Venison Stew. Additional protein, such as more turkey ham instead of bacon, could make it into a standalone meal salad, especially for PT. CT's could pair it with a Curried Peanut Soup or Miso Soup with Watercress for a satisfying meal.

1 wash and chop broccoli heads and peeled, tender parts of stems into large mixing or serving bowl. Mix with minced red onion and minced dried cranberries.

2 sauté turkey bacon strips over medium heat in 8" skillet until crisp, but not burnt. Remove and crumble over broccoli.

3 mix mayonnaise and yogurt together in measuring cup. Pour over salad. Toss to mix. Mix in chopped walnuts. Serve.

Serves 4. Preparation time: 15 minutes.

Quick Crunchy 'Cado

A nice combination of creamy, cool, and crunchy.

1½   cups cucumber, peeled, seeded and diced

1½   cups celery, chunky cuts

1   med avocado, pitted and cubed

½   cup dill pickle gherkins, chopped

½   cup flat-leaf Italian parsley, loosely packed

1   tsp lime juice

½   tsp Spike vegetable seasoning or Mrs Dash

5–6   grinds freshly ground black pepper

4   leaf lettuce leaves

¼   cup black olive slices

1 place cut up cucumber, celery, avocado, and dill pickles in large mixing or serving bowl. Vegetable cuts for this recipe should be roughly equal, about ½" each.

2 roughly chop flat-leaf parsley. Stir into salad ingredients.

3 pour lime juice over salad and stir lightly. Add vegetable seasoning and pepper. Stir lightly to mix, being careful not to smash avocado pieces. Serve immediately with leaf lettuce leaves and black olive garnish.

Serves 2. Preparation time: 10 minutes.

Nutrition Facts

	calories	total fat	carbs	protein
Mixed Type:	183	14g	15g	4g
Carb Type:	108	7g	11g	3g
Protein Type:	181	14g	15g	4g

Cooking Tips

PT: Increase celery to 2 cups and use only 1 cup diced cucumber.

CT: Increase cucumber to 2¼ cups and use only ¾ cup celery. Use ½ avocado, blending it with lime juice, vegetable seasoning, and 2 Tbsp of water for a smooth avocado dressing.

Notes and Suggestions

This is more of a PT kind of salad with its creamy chunks of avocado. Squares of provolone and/or 4 oz of turkey ham per serving could turn this into a meal salad for all types.

Sea Salad

Brimming with important trace minerals your body likely needs, this unusual looking Asian-inspired recipe will kick up the flavor and nutrition of your mini-meals.

2	lbs mixed spring greens
1½	cups Sea Salad Side (page 246)
¼	cup Savory Sunny Seed Mix (page 215)

Nutrition Facts

	calories	total fat	carbs	protein
Mixed Type:	156	8g	18g	69g
Carb Type:	76	4g	9g	4g
Protein Type:	176	11g	16g	8g

Cooking Tips

PT: Can double seed mix. You may find you want to add another tablespoon of oil for more satiety. Substitute spinach for part of the mixed greens.

CT: Reduce the seed mix to 2 Tbsp, sprinkled on top of the salad, or use a few sprinkles (1 tsp) of Sunny Seed Gomasio, instead.

Notes and Suggestions

This is a nutrient-rich salad that could be served with an Oriental-style dish, such as Ostrich Stir-Fry, if you are a CT, or even Hot Wings, Thighs & Things, or Miso Glazed Salmon for Protein types.

1 wash and drain spring greens, if not already pre-washed. Divide salad onto individual serving plates or serving bowl.

2 top with Sea Salad Side mixture, pouring juice over top as dressing.

3 serve as is, or sprinkled with Savory Sunny Seed Mix, if desired. Serve immediately.

Serves 4. Preparation time: 5 minutes.

Spinach Salad

Spinach and mushrooms, two of the Protein Type's most recommended vegetables, coexist happily in this popular salad with a savory seed topping.

2	10 oz bags fresh baby spinach leaves, washed and stemmed or greens for CT (see cooking tips below)
8	oz button mushrooms, sliced
½	med cucumber, peeled, seeded and sliced
4	eggs, semi-hardcooked, halved
2	Tbsp Savory Sunny Seed Mix (page 215)
2	Tbsp Basic Herb Vinaigrette or Sunny Seed Salad Dressing (page 237)

1 drain spinach and pat dry with paper towels or spin dry in salad spinner. Place in serving bowl or on individual salad plates.

2 arrange mushrooms, cucumber slices, and egg halves on salad. Top with Savory Sunny Seed Mix and Basic Herb Vinaigrette or Sunny Seed Salad Dressing.

Serves 4. Preparation time: 5 minutes.

Nutrition Facts

	calories	*total fat*	*carbs*	*protein*
Mixed Type:	157	9g	10g	13g
Carb Type:	123	7g	7g	9g
Protein Type:	178	10g	11g	14g

Cooking Tips

PT: Can increase seed mix to ¼ cup and double the mushrooms. Substitute celery for cucumber, if desired.

CT: Since spinach is not one of your highly recommended greens, replace at least half of the spinach with a mixture of bok choy, Napa cabbage, parsley, watercress or other greens. Increase cucumbers to 2. Top with Basic Herb Vinaigrette. Skip seed mix and add ½ cup mung bean sprouts.

Notes and Suggestions

This is an ideal salad for a PT. Make it into a meal salad by increasing the eggs and adding turkey bacon bits. Or serve with Herb Seasoned Broiled Steak, Horseradish Buffalo Burgers, or Mustard Tarragon Salmon for a delicious, satisfying meal.

Stuffed Cukes and Zukes

A versatile little recipe that goes as appetizer, snack or salad to the next potluck, when you don't know what to do with all those cucumbers and zucchinis in your garden.

8	baby zucchini
8	small cucumbers
¾	cup Sesame Miso Spread (page 221)
½	cup chopped curly parsley

1 wash zucchinis and cucumbers and cut in half lengthwise. Scoop out seeds with melon baller or small measuring spoon. Discard or put through juicer.

2 shred two of the baby zucchinis on the larger holes of a vegetable grater. Gently pat dry with paper towel and place in small bowl.

3 add chopped parsley and sesame spread to shredded zucchini and mix together until combined.

4 pile vegetable filling into zucchini and cucumber halves. Arrange on platter, decorate with parsley sprigs and allow 2 "boats" per person.

Serves 8. Preparation time: 15 minutes.

Nutrition Facts

	calories	total fat	carbs	protein
Mixed Type:	160	12g	11g	5g
Carb Type:	139	10g	10g	5g
Protein Type:	189	16g	8g	6g

Cooking Tips

PT: Could use half celery stalks instead of cucumbers. Increase Sesame Miso Spread to 1 cup.

CT: Reduce Sesame Spread to ½ cup and increase chopped parsley to 1 cup.

Notes and Suggestions

These vegetable-stuffed vegetables make a great CT platter. Just reduce the amount of seeds, or use hummus bean spread instead of sesame spread. Serve as an appetizer, counted as a vegetable or salad, for part of your balanced meal. PT's will probably want to add more protein to feel satisfied, but this can be a great carry-along snack, as well.

Sunny Rainbow Cabbage Salad

*This coleslaw plus is not only beautiful, it's a winner in the flavor depart-
ment, one of those cold weather salads you'll use again and again.*

2	cups shredded green cabbage
1	cup shredded red cabbage
1/2	cup finely shredded carrots
2/3	cup parsley, chopped
1	med scallion, chopped
2	Tbsp grapeseed oil
2	Tbsp apple cider vinegar
1	tsp dill weed
1	tsp Spike vegetable seasoning or Mrs.Dash
2	Tbsp Savory Sunny Seed Mix (page 215)

1 in large serving bowl, combine cabbages, carrots, parsley, and scallion.

2 combine oil, vinegar, dill weed, and vegetable seasoning. Pour over salad. Sprinkle with seed mix and toss well.

3 flavor is improved, if refrigerated for at least 20 minutes before serving.

Serves 4. Preparation time: 15 minutes.

Nutrition Facts

	calories	total fat	carbs	protein
Mixed Type:	116	9g	8g	3g
Carb Type:	90	6g	10g	3g
Protein Type:	165	14g	3g	4g

Cooking Tips

PT: You can substitute 1 cup of spinach for 1 cup of the green cabbage, add 1/2 cup finely sliced celery, and decrease red cabbage to 1/2 cup. Increase seed mix to 1/4 cup and oil to 3 Tbsp.

CT: Add 1 large zucchini, shredded. Use 1 1/2 Tbsp grapeseed oil. Reduce seed mix to 1 Tbsp or use 2 tsp Sunny Seed Gomasio, sprinkled on top.

Notes and Suggestions

A rainbow of colors and flavors, this salad is a way to spark up winter meals and appetites. Add a bit of toasted sesame oil for an Oriental flavor. Pair this with a stew, chili or Hot Wings for a satisfying meal for game night. Or serve it as the salad side in a tailgate picnic basket with cold, oven "fried" chicken breast.

Watercress Salad

A delightful spring-into-summer salad that goes well with almost any salmon or light chicken dish.

3	Tbsp fresh lemon juice
2	tsp Dijon mustard
2	Tbsp extra virgin olive oil
1/2	tsp tamari soy sauce
2	grinds fresh black pepper
3	bunches watercress, washed and stemmed
1	cup jicama, peeled, cut into sticks
2	Tbsp slivered almonds, toasted
2	Tbsp feta cheese, crumbled

Nutrition Facts

	calories	total fat	carbs	protein
Mixed Type:	134	10g	8g	4g
Carb Type:	126	9g	10g	3g
Protein Type:	235	22g	6g	7g

Cooking Tips

PT: Can add 2 cups torn spinach and 1 cup asparagus cuts to make this salad more in line with your type. Increase oil to 1/4 cup. Use 2/3 cup jicama sticks. Increase nuts to 3 Tbsp and feta cheese to 3 oz.

CT: Can increase jicama to 1 1/2 cups. Reduce oil to 1 Tbsp. Reduce or eliminate almonds and substitute sliced waterchestnuts.

Notes and Suggestions

A delightful salad that goes well with almost any salmon or light chicken dish. A meal for any type, but especially PT.

1 in jar or glass measuring cup, combine lemon juice, mustard, olive oil, tamari, and pepper. Whisk to blend.

2 wash and stem watercress. Place in large serving bowl. Drizzle on desired amount of salad dressing and lightly toss to coat.

3 divide salad onto serving plates. Top with jicama sticks, almonds, and feta cheese. Serve immediately.

Serves 4. Preparation time: 10 minutes.

THE RECIPES: Vegetables

Low in calories and fat, high in fiber, and with almost all the vitamins and minerals your body needs, vegetables are the nutritional goldmine of all foods. Fortunately, there is a wide diversity of vegetables available, and the recipes in this cookbook make great use of them, especially the lower carbohydrate, non-starchy, above-ground vegetables recommended for your metabolic type.

You'll find yourself using vegetables in some unexpected ways with these recipes. In addition to one-dish meals like stews, soups and salads, you'll also find new and interesting recipes for sprouted snack vegetables made from beans and seeds, fermented vegetables like sauerkraut, and nutritious sea and land vegetable combos. You'll find juiced and puréed vegetables made into beverages, and dehydrated into Vegetable Leathers and No-Grain Vegetable Crisper crackers for tasty snacks. You'll even find no-grain wrappers for sandwiches and roll-ups, made primarily from vegetables.

With the tools and recipes in this book, you will not only be able to eat your veggies—you will really enjoy them as lifelong partners in helping you achieve total health and well-being.

Braised Brazilian Greens

When flash-seared in a wok or heavy skillet instead of being cooked to death in water, dark leafy greens like collards, kale, or swiss chard become a whole new eating experience—and retain their nutrients.

3	lbs collard greens, kale, turnip greens, bok choy, Swiss chard or mixture of dark leafy greens
2	Tbsp coconut oil
7	cloves fresh garlic, chopped
6	oz turkey ham, diced
¼	cup clean, filtered water
1	Tbsp tamari soy sauce
4	grinds fresh black pepper
2-3	dashes hot pepper sauce

Nutrition Facts

	calories	total fat	carbs	protein
Mixed Type:	186	9g	17g	14g
Carb Type:	111	4g	16g	8g
Protein Type:	278	14g	21g	22g

Cooking Tips

PT: Substitute 2 lbs spinach and use only 1 lb of the other greens. Increase turkey ham to 10 ounces.

CT: Reduce coconut oil to 1 Tbsp. Omit or reduce turkey ham to 3 oz, if combining this dish with another vegetable for a whole meal. Could also used semi-hardcooked eggs as protein.

Notes and Suggestions

This is a quick and easy standalone meal or mini-meal for fall or winter, when dark leafy greens are plentiful. This can be paired with dark meat turkey cutlets or a bison meatloaf for a PT meal. CT's could use it with Crunchy Chicken Casserole, white meat Roast Chicken, Ostrich Meatballs. Or add 2–3 oz of turkey ham cut into matchsticks and another vegetable such as Sautéed Cabbage with Dill.

1 wash greens. Cut along middle to remove woody stems.

2 cut into chiffonade or thin strips by rolling stacked green leaves lengthwise into a roll and cutting crosswise into ¼" strips.

3 heat a large wok or deep heavy skillet with cover over high heat. When hot, add oil and garlic, and sauté for 30–45 seconds or until starting to brown lightly. Add turkey ham and sauté for 1 more minute.

4 add cut up greens and stir-fry over high heat, stirring constantly for about a minute. Add water, cover and steam for about 2 minutes.

5 add seasonings and taste. Serve immediately as a side dish or on its own as a satisfying mini-meal.

Serves 4. Preparation time: 10 minutes.

Broccoli-in-a-Hurry Curry

Almost everyone likes this simple, yet slightly exotic-tasting vegetable dish. Fast, easy, and elegant, even if you're preparing for a special gathering or entertaining.

| 1 | head broccoli |
| 1/3 | cup Curry Mayonnaise (page 238) |

1 wash broccoli and cut off woody ends. Cut broccoli into spears.

2 steam broccoli over boiling water in a steamer basket or colander for 7 or so minutes until bright

3 spoon Curry Mayonnaise over hot broccoli in serving dish or serve on the side. Serve immediately.

Serves 4. Preparation time: 10 minutes.

Nutrition Facts

	calories	total fat	carbs	protein
Mixed Type:	184	15g	10g	5g
Carb Type:	140	10g	10g	5g
Protein Type:	228	20g	10g	5g

Cooking Tips

PT: Use 1/2 cup Curry Dressing.

CT: Use 1/4 cup reduced fat Curry Dressing (use 1/2 lowfat yogurt and 1/2 mayonnaise).

Notes and Suggestions

This simple, yet dressy vegetable dish can complete a primarily meat-based entrée such as Grilled Caribbean Chicken, Roast Chicken, or Turkey, or even a plain meat or seafood dish such as Broiled Miso Salmon or Herb Seasoned Steak Broil for a PT. CT eaters can use the reduced fat version of the Curry Dressing and enjoy the dish combined with a soup, meat, and vegetable salad or casserole for a complete repast.

Broiled Eggplant Parmish

This Eggplant "Parmesan-ish" vegetable dish has the taste of the authentic version, but is ready in a fraction of the time, with a fraction of the carbs.

1	med eggplant, cut on an angle into 1/4" slices
1	Tbsp extra virgin olive oil
1	tsp sea salt
1	Tbsp poultry seasoning
2	tsp dried oregano or basil
2	med tomatoes, thinly sliced
4	Tbsp Basil Pesto (page 239)
1/4	cup grated Parmesan cheese

Nutrition Facts

	calories	total fat	carbs	protein
Mixed Type:	106	6g	12g	5g
Carb Type:	90	5g	11g	3g

Cooking Tips

PT: Eggplant is not really a PT type of vegetable, so you'll probably want to skip this dish.

CT: Reduce the pesto and Parmesan cheese to 2 Tbsp each for the whole recipe.

Notes and Suggestions

This could be served as a vegetable side dish with a Marinated Italian Salad, Fresh Mozzarella Plate, or Fennel Parmesan and a salad. Or increase portion size by serving to 2 only, and serve with Horseradish Buffalo.

1 turn on broiler. Brush or spray eggplant slices lightly on both sides with oil. Sprinkle with salt, poultry seasoning, and oregano or basil leaves.

2 broil eggplant slices for 3–4 minutes on each side, until they start to brown.

3 remove from oven. Place a thin slice of tomato on each eggplant slice and spread with Basil Pesto.

4 sprinkle grated Parmesan cheese over top and broil for 1–2 more minutes until warmed through, and pesto and cheese start to bubble. Serve immediately.

Serves 4. Preparation time: 15 minutes.

Brussels Sprouts Trio

These quickly braised "little cabbages" join kale and leeks in a vegetable side laced with country Dijon mustard.

2	**Tbsp coconut oil**
2	**med garlic cloves, smashed**
2	**med leeks, washed and sliced**
4	**cups Brussels sprouts, washed, stemmed and quartered**
1	**tsp fresh or 1½ tsp dried rosemary**
1	**bunch kale, stems removed, coarsely chopped**
¼	**cup water**
3	**Tbsp Dijon or country Dijon mustard**

1 heat a wok or deep, heavy porcelain-clad pan with a cover over high heat.

2 add oil and garlic, stir for a few seconds. Then add leek slices. Stir-fry, stirring constantly, for about 2–3 minutes or until leeks start to wilt.

3 add Brussels sprouts and rosemary and stir-fry for 2–3 minutes. Reduce heat to medium, add cut up kale and water, stirring to combine. Cover and steam for 3–5 minutes, until fork tender.

4 remove cover, stir in Dijon mustard to coat. Remove to serving dish and serve immediately.

Serves 4. Preparation time: 10 minutes.

Nutrition Facts

	calories	total fat	carbs	protein
Mixed Type:	163	8g	21g	6g
Carb Type:	133	5g	21g	6g
Protein Type:	149	8g	8g	6g

Cooking Tips

PT: Adapt this more to your type by substituting spinach for kale, using half green beans and half Brussels sprouts, added at the same time.

CT: Reduce oil to 1 Tbsp.

Notes and Suggestions

This fast, cold season vegetable could be made into a mini-meal by serving it with sliced turkey ham, Beef 'n Beer Stew or Ground Turkey and Gravy on a frosty, midwinter evening.

Cauliflower with Tapenade Crown

A simple, yet elegant steamed cauliflower with an olive tapenade or olive-nut paste crown. Sounds more complicated than it really is, yet looks beautiful with cauliflowerettes reassembled to look like a whole head on its own original leafy base "plate."

1	head cauliflower, about 2 pounds
4	Tbsp Black Olive Tapenade (page 240)

Nutrition Facts

	calories	total fat	carbs	protein
Mixed Type:	113	4g	17g	5g
Protein Type:	173	8	23g	8g

Cooking Tips

PT: This is an ideal PT vegetable dish. Double the amount of black olive-nut paste.

CT: Broccoli, cabbage, turnip or summer squash could be substituted for the cauliflower. Try a small portion of the Tapenade, but if you find it's too rich, you could also try a Basil Pesto (page 239) or Red Onion Cilantro Relish (page 245) topping instead.

Notes and Suggestions

Another vegetable that's sophisticated enough to serve for company or as an extra special family meal. You don't have to fuss with the presentation, if you don't want to. Pair this with Roast Chicken, Grilled Bison Steaks, or Mustard Tarragon Salmon.

1 place a steamer basket or strainer into the bottom of a large covered kettle. Add 1–2" of water and bring to a boil.

2 working from the back of the cauliflower head, remove leaves and stem in one piece by pulling back leaves and cutting stem through at the base of the head. Place base plate on platter or flat serving dish.

3 being careful and using a sharp knife, break cauliflower into 2–3" flowerettes, cutting deep gashes in stems to shorten cooking time.

4 steam cauliflowerettes over boiling water on medium high, until barely tender, for approximately 8–9 minutes. Remove from heat.

5 reassemble cauliflowerettes to look like original head on top of their leaves on platter. Spread or mound olive tapenade over top and serve. Or serve accompanied by a small bowl of the rich olive-nut paste.

6 if you have the luxury of more time, this can be prepared by steaming the whole head of cauliflower intact as above. Or rub with extra virgin olive oil, sprinkle with sea salt and roast in 350°F oven, 35–40 minutes, covering with tapenade the last five minutes, for a more flavorful dish.

Serves 4. Preparation time: 15 minutes.

Confetti Spaghetti Squash Sauté

This brightly colored red, yellow, and green vegetable dish is beautiful enough for company, quick enough for everyday.

1	**large spaghetti squash, cooked and scooped out of shell**
2	**Tbsp raw or organic butter**
1	**med shallot, minced**
2	**Tbsp red pepper, finely chopped**
2	**Tbsp green bell pepper, finely chopped**
½	**tsp Spike vegetable seasoning or Mrs. Dash**
	freshly ground black pepper to taste

1 if not already cooked, boil spaghetti squash, cut in half, in large pan with water over medium heat until fork tender. Remove from pan, cool slightly and scoop out spaghetti strands with fork.

2 in large pan, melt butter over medium heat and add minced shallot. Sauté lightly for about a minute until flavors are released.

3 add cooked spaghetti squash and stir to mix. Stir in chopped red and green peppers. Add seasonings to taste and continue cooking until vegetable is heated through, about 2–3 minutes.

4 remove to serving bowl. Garnish with Savory Sunny Seed Mix, Sunny Seed Gomasio or Parmesan cheese, as desired.

Serves 4. Preparation time: 10 minutes.

Nutrition Facts

	calories	total fat	carbs	protein
Mixed Type:	156	7g	24g	3g
Carb Type:	130	4g	24g	3g
Protein Type:	156	7g	24g	3g

Cooking Tips

PT: This is not your best recipe, unless you serve a minimum ½ cup as a base for No-Pasta Primavera Vegetables, and add protein like meat balls or Ground Turkey and Gravy.

CT: Reduce butter to 1 Tbsp.

Notes and Suggestions

Serve this, if you are MX or CT eater, with a fresh tomato sauce and lowfat Parmesan cheese and lean, ground, seasoned ostrich as a standalone recipe for a quick and easy weeknight meal.

Fennel Parmesan

A tasty accompaniment for fish, chicken or lamb.

2	lb fennel, washed and diagonally-sliced
1	cup clean, filtered water
2	tsp raw or organic butter
1/2	tsp sea salt
5–6	grinds freshly ground black pepper
2/3	cup Parmesan or Romano cheese

1 heat large skillet over medium heat. Add fennel slices and water. Steam fennel for 5 minutes, until water is evaporated.

2 when water is gone, melt butter in skillet. Stir fennel to coat and cook 2–3 minutes more.

3 Sprinkle on salt, pepper and Parmesan cheese. Heat for 2–3 more minutes or place under broiler, until cheese starts to turn golden. Serve immediately.

Serves 4. Preparation time: 15 minutes.

Nutrition Facts

	calories	total fat	carbs	protein
Mixed Type:	125	7g	9g	8g
Carb Type:	90	4g	11g	4g
Protein Type:	133	8g	8g	10g

Cooking Tips

PT: While fennel is not one of your highly recommended vegetables, you might try this recipe with a whole head of celery and half a bunch of asparagus spears, sprinkled with 1/2 tsp Spike vegetable seasoning or Mrs. Dash before cooking. Use 3/4 cup Parmesan cheese.

CT: Reduce Parmesan cheese to 1/3 cup reduced fat cheese.

Notes and Suggestions

Serve Fennel Parmesan as a special vegetable side dish to accompany a Broiled Lemon Fish or Roast Chicken dinner, paired with a mixed greens and radicchio salad tossed with Dijon vinaigrette dressing.

Gado Gado Vegetables

This Indonesian favorite with its peanut buttery sauce does an amazing job of transforming common, everyday vegetables into downright good eating.

1	med head cabbage, cut into wedges
2	med turnips, peeled and cut into 8 slices
3	stalks celery
1	cup green beans
1/3	cup Asian Dressing made with peanut butter (page 236)

1 bring 1 cup water to boil in bottom of large, covered saucepan.

2 place vegetables in steamer basket and lower into pan. Cover and steam for 5–8 minutes or until vegetables are tender.

3 remove to serving bowl and pour Asian Dressing on top. Serve immediately.

Serves 4. Preparation time: 15 minutes.

Nutrition Facts

	calories	total fat	carbs	protein
Mixed Type:	193	10g	25g	8g
Carb Type:	157	7g	23g	7g
Protein Type:	217	13g	23g	9g

Cooking Tips

PT: Reduce cabbage to 1/2 head. Increase celery to 5 large stalks and green beans to 2 cups. Could also add 2 cups spinach leaves. Increase dressing to 1/2 cup.

CT: Reduce dressing to 1/4 cup.

Notes and Suggestions

This is a classic vegetable main dish that could stand on its own for an MX or CT winter meal. PT's will want to add some protein in the form of turkey ham or bison summer sausage chunks. Or serve as a vegetable side dish with a heavier meat entrée such as Turkey Cutlets or even roast beef.

Grecian Spinach

This spinach with Greek flair is easy to make as an everyday vegetable on its own, or as a special dinner partner for lamb, chicken or fish.

1	Tbsp coconut oil
1/2	small red onion, thin sliced into rings
2	lb fresh baby spinach, washed and stemmed
1/2	tsp grated lemon peel
1/2	tsp sea salt
3–4	grinds freshly ground black pepper
1/4	cup feta cheese, crumbled

Nutrition Facts

	calories	total fat	carbs	protein
Mixed Type:	111	6g	10g	8g
Carb Type:	89	4g	12g	7g
Protein Type:	134	8g	10g	9g

Cooking Tips

PT: Increase feta cheese to 1/2 cup.

CT: Decrease oil to 1 Tbsp. Decrease spinach to 1 lb. Add 1 1/2 lbs other dark leafy greens such as chard or beet greens. Increase lemon peel to 1 tsp. For cheese, use 1 Tbsp feta mixed with 1 Tbsp nonfat cottage cheese.

Notes and Suggestions

This recipe is ideal for PT, but can be modified for CT by adding other dark leafy greens such as Swiss chard or beet greens. To make this into a meal, add protein such as turkey ham or bacon for a PT or MX. CT can increase the proportion of lowfat cottage cheese. Serve this vegetable with Herbed Lemony Lamb Chops or Chicken Breast. If you find that your thirst increases or you feel strange after eating this quantity of spinach, try increasing the proportion of the other greens (except PT) and drink more clean water.

1 heat a large pan with a lid over medium high heat. Add oil and sliced red onion. Sauté until onion starts to wilt.

2 add spinach and quickly sauté for 2–3 minutes. Add lemon peel, salt and pepper. Cook a few seconds more to release flavors.

3 add crumbled feta cheese and stir to incorporate. Transfer to serving dish and serve immediately.

Serves 4. Preparation time: 10 minutes.

Green Bean Casserole

Yes, you can have your traditional holiday favorite, modified with alternative crunchy toppings.

1	lb fresh green beans, washed, snapped and cut up
½	lb fresh mushrooms, sliced
1	11 oz can organic cream of mushroom soup
2	Tbsp grated horseradish
1	tsp Worcestershire sauce
3	grinds fresh ground black pepper
½	cup broken Vegetable Crispers (page 223) or
3	Tbsp Savory Sunny Seed Mix

1 preheat oven to 350° F. Combine all ingredients except toppings together in oiled casserole. Cover.

2 bake for about 45 minutes until beans are tender. Remove cover and sprinkle with topping of choice. Return to oven for ten more minutes, increasing heat to Broil, and broiling top, if desired.

3 this dish can be made quickly for everyday consumption, by steaming the green beans and mushrooms over boiling water in a steamer basket or colander for 8–9 minutes. Reserve water for soup stock.

4 stir soup, horseradish, Worcestershire sauce, and pepper into beans. Return to burner and heat through, approx 3 minutes. Transfer to serving dish and sprinkle with desired toppings.

Serves 4. Preparation time: 10 minutes.

Nutrition Facts

	calories	total fat	carbs	protein
Mixed Type:	118	5g	16g	5g
Protein Type:	125	5g	17g	6g

Cooking Tips

PT: You'll be happy to know this is just your type of vegetable dish. You can even increase mushrooms to a 12 oz pkg. You can choose the Savory Sunny Seed Mix topper or use both toppings!

CT: Even though green beans are not your most recommended vegetable, you can enjoy this as a special treat, following the recipe as listed.

Notes and Suggestions

More than likely, you'll be inclined to serve this with a traditional Thanksgiving or Christmas spread, but you could also make this into a whole meal casserole by adding leftover, cooked dark meat chicken or turkey, pieces of roast beef or even leftover chunks of meat loaf or Quick Beef Steaks with Wine, if you are a PT or MX.

Lemon Pepper Green Beans

An easy, fresh green bean side dish you could serve to guests or at any weekday dinner, substituting Lemon Pepper seasoning, if you are in a hurry.

3	lb fresh green beans
2	Tbsp organic butter or coconut oil
2	cloves garlic, minced
¼	cup lemon juice
2	tsp grated lemon rind or 2–3 drops lemon oil
	freshly grated black pepper
2	tsp Spike vegetable seasoning or Mrs. Dash

Nutrition Facts

	calories	total fat	carbs	protein
Mixed Type:	174	7g	27g	6g
Protein Type:	234	14g	27g	6g

Cooking Tips

PT: Definitely a PT vegetable dish. You can use coconut oil or butter, increasing to 2 Tbsp.

CT: Instead of green beans, you could make the same dish with broccoli, zucchini or summer squash, Brussels sprouts or dark leafy greens.

Notes and Suggestions

This peppery vegetable would be a good accompaniment to a saucy meat dish like Turkey and Gravy or Crockpot Chicken Curry for all types.

1 in large heavy skillet over high heat, stir-fry green beans in butter or coconut oil and garlic until crisp tender.

2 reduce heat to medium, add lemon juice, lemon peel, pepper, and vegetable seasoning. Cover and let steam for 2–3 minutes, stirring occasionally.

3 transfer to serving bowl and serve immediately

Serves 4. Preparation time: 10 minutes.

Mashed Fotatoes

You might be surprised how much this "like mashed potatoes" dish simulates the taste and texture of the "real" thing.

1	head fresh cauliflower, about 1¹/₂ lbs
2	Tbsp organic or raw butter
¹/₄	cup organic or raw half and half
¹/₄	tsp sea salt
2–3	grinds black pepper

1 steam cauliflower until tender in steamer basket or small amount of water in saucepan.

2 in food processor, blend cauliflower, butter, cream, sea salt and pepper, until smooth.

3 transfer to serving bowl. Serve immediately.

Serves 4. Preparation time: 15 minutes.

Nutrition Facts

	calories	*total fat*	*carbs*	*protein*
Mixed Type:	163	8g	20g	8g
Carb Type:	138	4g	23g	9g
Protein Type:	214	14g	20g	8g

Cooking Tips

PT: This creamy dish is right for your type. You can increase the butter to ¹/₄ cup.

CT: You will want to substitute lowfat buttermilk for the cream and reduce the butter to 1 Tbsp.

Notes and Suggestions

This is an amazingly authentic substitute for those high starchy spuds, especially when served as a holiday vegetable or base for meat with gravy like Ground Turkey and Gravy or Red Peppery Buffalo Steaks.

No-Pasta Primavera Vegetables

This classic Italian vegetable mélange can be prepared as a side dish, or ladled over spaghetti squash, Zucchetti or low-carb pasta for a wonderful meal anytime.

2	med zucchini, sliced
2	med yellow squash, sliced
3	stalks celery, diagonally sliced
1	small red pepper, seeded, cut into strips
1	small yellow pepper, seeded, cut into strips
1	cup broccoli flowerettes
3	Tbsp extra virgin olive oil
3–4	cloves garlic, sliced
1	cup fresh basil leaves, packed, or 3 Tbsp dried
1	cup Italian flat-leaf parsley
3	Tbsp tamari soy sauce
1/4	cup Parmesan cheese
3	Tbsp Savory Sunny Seed Mix, optional (page 215)

Nutrition Facts

	calories	total fat	carbs	protein
Mixed Type:	205	3g	18g	9g
Carb Type:	171	9g	17g	9g
Protein Type:	250	17g	19g	11g

Cooking Tips

PT: Omit yellow peppers. Substitute 2 cups asparagus for zucchini, 1 cup green beans for broccoli, increase celery to 5 stalks. Add 1 more Tbsp oil and increase seed mix and Parmesan cheese to 1/3 cup.

CT: Follow recipe as is or vary by omitting celery and increasing broccoli to 2 cups. Reduce oil and Parmesan cheese to 2 Tbsp. Omit seeds.

Notes and Suggestions

The co-author's quick, prize-winning recipe, adapted from the classic Italian dish, is a staple that you probably will find yourself using regularly, varying with vegetables in season and adding different protein foods, such as dark meat of chicken, turkey, beef or fish for PT eaters. It could stand on its own as a main meal for CT or MX, but could also work with ostrich or chicken breast. Add chunks of uncooked meat with the garlic or add leftover cooked meat at the end.

1 wash and cut up vegetables. Once you master this recipe, you'll be able to cut up the vegetables while the pan is heating.

2 heat one large, heavy, porcelain-clad Dutch oven or wok over high heat. Add olive oil and garlic slices. Stir-fry 1–2 minutes.

3 add zucchini, yellow squash, celery, broccoli, and stir-fry, stirring constantly, for 7–8 minutes until vegetables start to soften and brighten.

4 add red and yellow pepper strips, basil leaves, and parsley and 2/3 cup water. Cover. Reduce heat to medium high and steam 3–4 minutes.

5 remove from heat. Add tamari soy sauce and stir. Serve immediately as is, or sprinkled with Parmesan cheese and a sprinkle of Savory Sunny Seed Mix, if desired.

Serves 4. Preparation time: 15 minutes.

Roasted Asparagus

This is a delicious vegetable, quickly roasted in a pan or slow-roasted in the oven.

2	lb fresh asparagus
3	Tbsp coconut oil or organic or raw butter
1	Tbsp Bragg's Liquid Aminos or tamari soy sauce

1 if oven roasting, preheat oven to 500°F. Wash, pat dry and cut off woody ends of fresh asparagus.

2 mix coconut oil and Bragg's in frying or baking pan. Roll asparagus around in oil mixture to coat.

3 roast on stovetop for 7–9 minutes over medium heat, shaking pan several times to prevent sticking. Or bake at 500° for 8–10 minutes, stirring occasionally. Serve.

Serves 4. Preparation time: 15 minutes.

Nutrition Facts

	calories	total fat	carbs	protein
Mixed Type:	124	9g	9g	6g
Protein Type:	169	14g	9g	5g

Cooking Tips

PT: Another optimum PT vegetable. Increase oil or butter to 4 Tbsp.

CT: Vary the recipe by using other vegetables, including turnips, okra, cabbage chunks or baby onions, but decrease oil to 1 Tbsp or less.

Notes and Suggestions

If you have the time for a special treat or family dinner, you will LOVE slow roasted asparagus. Simply follow the recipe, but roast marinated asparagus at 250°F. for 6–7 hours, stirring occasionally. Melts in your mouth!

Sautéed Cabbage with Dill

Once again, cole crops like cabbage and turnips are delicious when lightly sautéed instead of boiled. The double dose of dill really perks up this normally mundane vegetable.

2	Tbsp organic butter or coconut oil
1	med head green cabbage, cut into 1/2–3/4" pieces
1	tsp dill seeds
1/2	tsp sea salt or Spike vegetable seasoning
4–5	grinds fresh black pepper
2	tsp dried dill weed

Nutrition Facts

	calories	total fat	carbs	protein
Mixed Type:	111	6g	14g	4g
Carb Type:	85	3g	14g	4g

Cooking Tips

PT: Not an ideal vegetable for your type. Try this recipe with 2 lbs green beans or asparagus.

CT: Reduce the butter or oil to 1 Tbsp.

Notes and Suggestions

Cabbage can be delicious served this way as a vegetable side dish with a hearty soup or stew, or as the complement to a small portion of roasted Cornish hen or breast of chicken stir-fry.

1 heat butter or coconut oil in large skillet over medium heat.

2 add cabbage chunks and dill seeds. Sauté cabbage over medium high, stirring frequently, until cabbage is translucent and starts to wilt, approximately 6–7 minutes. Okay if it gets a little browned.

3 remove from heat, Stir in sea salt, fresh black pepper and dill weed. Serve immediately.

Serves 4. Preparation time: 10 minutes.

Savory Summer Squash

One of the simplest, yet most delightful summer vegetable dishes, this is a great "what to do with" recipe for a bumper crop of garden squash.

4	large crookneck yellow squash
2	Tbsp raw or organic butter
2	cloves fresh garlic, smashed
½	tsp Spike vegetable seasoning or Mrs. Dash

1 wash and cut up yellow squash into ½" pieces. Discard any big seeds or put through juicer..

2 heat medium skillet over medium heat. Melt butter and add smashed garlic.

3 add squash and stir to coat. Cover and simmer for 5–7 minutes.

4 sprinkle with vegetable seasoning. Serve immediately.

Serves 4. Preparation time: 10 minutes.

Nutrition Facts

	calories	total fat	carbs	protein
Mixed Type:	105	6g	11g	4g
Carb Type:	80	3g	11g	4g
Protein Type:	115	6g	13g	6g

Cooking Tips

PT: Substitute half asparagus cuts and cook the same way. It's OK if you find you need to double your portions.

CT: Reduce the butter to 1 Tbsp.

Notes and Suggestions

When summer squash or zucchini is cooked in this way, it appeals to everyone, even small children, as long as it's not over-cooked. Pair it with a green salad and low-fat cottage or farmer's cheese on a hot night for a CT, or team it with a heartier Crunchy Chicken Salad or burgers on the grill for an MX or PT.

Zesty Fennel with Pea Pods

This quick, unique vegetable combo takes on a new kick with a smoky bite of hot chipotle pepper sauce.

1½	Tbsp coconut oil
4	cups fennel, diagonally-sliced
2	Tbsp minced red onion or 1 sliced scallion
1	cup snow peas, cut in half on diagonal
1	tsp hot chipotle sauce or few dashes hot pepper sauce

1 heat medium skillet over medium heat.

2 add coconut oil, fennel and minced red onion. Steam-sauté, stirring frequently, for 5–6 minutes.

3 stir in snow peas. Cover, reduce heat and steam 3 minutes more.

4 add chipotle sauce and stir to coat. Serve immediately.

Serves 2. Preparation time: 10 minutes.

Nutrition Facts

	calories	total fat	carbs	protein
Mixed Type:	166	11g	17g	4g
Carb Type:	136	7g	17g	4g
Protein Type:	173	14g	11g	3g

Cooking Tips

PT: Fennel is not one of your highly recommended vegetables. You could, however, do a similar treatment with celery hearts instead. Use 2 Tbsp oil.

CT: Reduce oil to 1 Tbsp.

Notes and Suggestions

Excellent paired with Roasted Salmon (PT), Halibut or Tilapia (CT) with Pesto Crust. If you can't find the smoky chipotle pepper sauce, you could use a hot pepper sauce of your choice.

Zucchini with Walnuts

Another savory way to prepare this prolific garden vegetable.

3	**med zucchini squash**
¼	**cup raw or organic butter**
½	**tsp Spike vegetable seasoning or Mrs. Dash**
¼	**cup chopped organic walnuts**

1 wash zucchini. Cut off ends. Cut into ¼" slices.

2 heat a medium skillet over medium heat. Melt butter and add zucchini. Stir to coat.

3 sauté zucchini in butter, partially covered, for 7–8 minutes until translucent, but not soggy and limp.

4 remove from heat and transfer to serving bowl. Sprinkle with vegetable seasoning and chopped walnuts. Serve immediately.

Serves 4. Preparation time: 10 minutes.

Nutrition Facts

	calories	total fat	carbs	protein
Mixed Type:	174	17g	6g	3g
Carb Type:	107	9g	7g	3g
Protein Type:	195	18g	9g	5g

Cooking Tips

PT: While zucchinis are not on the top of the list of your best vegetables, you can vary this recipe with good results by decreasing quantity of squash to 2 and adding 1 lb asparagus cuts. You can increase butter to ⅓ cup.

CT: Add 1 more zucchini, but limit walnuts or other nuts to 1 Tbsp, finely chopped, and butter to 2 Tbsp.

Notes and Suggestions

This vegetable dish could be paired with a salad or soup and a little extra protein for a CT meal, but if it seems too "rich," decrease the butter or omit the nuts. Nuts and vegetables are a good combination for PT and MX, though, so you could enjoy this tasty vegetable side served with a protein main dish like Salmon Seviche or even heartier Red Peppery Buffalo Steaks or Herb Seasoned Steak Broil.

THE RECIPES: Soups

Soups can be eaten anytime, at any meal. The Japanese traditionally eat miso soup for breakfast, in contrast to most Westerners who usually only consider soup for lunch or as an appetizer for dinner. Soups are also easily convertible from a side dish to a more substantial main dish simply by adding a fourth- to a third-cup per serving of cooked concentrated protein, like leftover chicken, turkey, beef or bison, appropriate to your type.

When you take advantage of the batch cooking suggestions covered in the Chapter 10, you can really cut your time in the kitchen by planning at least one big pot of soup that you and your family can heat and eat anytime. One of the best insurance policies against snacking on high-sugar and high-starch snacks is having prepared foods, like soup, on hand for you and your family to grab.

Soups like Quick Miso Cup or Roasted Tomatillo Turkey Soup can be almost instantly prepared, while others can simmer long and slow, developing wonderful flavors in the crockpot. Either way, they pack a lot of nutrition into a small package. And since they don't require complicated techniques or multi-step procedures to prepare, they are a friend to new and seasoned cooks alike.

Artichoke & Asparagus Soup

A divine combination of some of the most heavenly vegetables and delicacies.

1	16 oz can artichoke hearts
1	Tbsp raw organic butter
1	med shallot or 2 small green onions, chopped
1	bunch asparagus, cut up
1	can water chestnuts, sliced
1	tsp Spike vegetable seasoning or Mrs. Dash
1	Tbsp fresh tarragon leaves or 1$^{1}/_{2}$ tsp dried
3	cups clean, filtered water or vegetable stock
$^{1}/_{4}$	cup raw macadamia nut butter or cashew butter
10	sprigs fresh watercress, broken

Nutrition Facts

	calories	*total fat*	*carbs*	*protein*
Mixed Type:	198	9g	27g	6g
Carb Type:	149	3g	28g	5g
Protein Type:	217	12g	27g	6g

Cooking Tips

PT: Increase nut butter to $^{1}/_{3}$ cup.

CT: Omit nut butter. Blend soup in blender until smooth.

Notes and Suggestions

To make this into a menu combo, try serving with a meal salad like Roasted Turkey Tomatillo Salad, Nouveau Salmon Nicoise, or for CT, Oriental Ostrich Salad.

1 pour liquid from artichoke hearts into saucepan. Chop artichokes coarsely and set aside.

2 into saucepan add butter, chopped shallot or onion, and asparagus cuts. Simmer gently for 4–5 minutes, until asparagus is fork tender.

3 add reserved artichokes, water chestnuts, vegetable seasoning and tarragon leaves. Heat through.

4 add about 2 cups water or stock to vegetables. Meanwhile, stir remaining cup water or stock gradually into nut butter until smooth, then carefully stir into soup. Stir soup frequently while heating over medium low until mixture is heated through. Do not boil.

5 taste for seasoning. Serve as is, or blend until smooth in blender. Ladle into serving bowls and garnish each with small sprigs of watercress.

Serves 4. Preparation time: 10 minutes.

Basic Vegetable Soup

A basic vegetable soup recipe that can be varied, depending upon your mood, the season, the allowable vegetables and seasonings you have on hand.

2	Tbsp raw or organic butter
2	med garlic cloves, smashed
½	cup chopped red onion
1	cup chopped celery
1	large carrot, diced
1	lb mushrooms, chopped
2	tsp dried thyme leaves
1	tsp dried marjoram leaves
1½	tsp sea salt
½	tsp black pepper
8	cups vegetable, chicken stock or water
1	Tbsp tamari soy sauce
1½	cups white wine, if desired
1	10 oz pkg snow peas
½	cup chopped parsley

1 heat a large, heavy skillet over medium heat. Add butter. When melted, add garlic and chopped onion. Sauté, stirring occasionally, until translucent, 3–5 minutes.

2 add celery, carrots, mushrooms, herbs, salt and pepper. Cover. Continue cooking, stirring occasionally, until vegetables are tender, roughly 7–8 minutes.

3 add stock or water, and wine, cover, and simmer for 10–20 minutes, more if you have time.

4 stir in tamari, wine, snow peas, and parsley. Simmer a few more minutes.

Serves 4. Preparation time: 25 minutes.

Nutrition Facts

	calories	total fat	carbs	protein
Mixed Type:	350	12g	30g	18g
Carb Type:	249	9g	27g	15g
Protein Type:	354	12g	30g	18g

Cooking Tips

PT: Add tenderloin, strip loin steak or chicken thigh pieces after sautéing the garlic for a fast version, or use chuck or stew meat for a longer simmering version. Increase celery to 2 cups.

CT: Follow the recipe as is or replace some of the mushrooms with zucchini chunks and broccoli or cut-up green or red peppers.

Notes and Suggestions

Soup recipes are usually more like guidelines, rather than strict formulas. Their beauty lies in their flexibility, economy and "meal in a bowl" potential. Cooks like them because of their ability to accommodate a wide range of vegetables and seasonings, whatever's on hand. It is wise to eat protein with this soup to make a balanced meal.

Blended Broccoli Soup

A deep green, quick and creamy blended soup that lets you "sneak in" other dark green leafy vegetables like kale, collards, turnip greens, Swiss chard, without detection. Don't overcook.

1	Tbsp coconut oil
2	med green onion, coarsely chopped
2	cloves garlic, minced
1	large head fresh broccoli, washed and chopped
1	Tbsp basil leaves, dried
2	cups chopped spinach, kale, turnip greens, collards, Swiss chard or other dark leafy greens
4	cups vegetable or chicken broth
2	cups coconut milk
1	tsp sea salt or kelp seaweed
2	dashes hot pepper sauce

Nutrition Facts

	calories	total fat	carbs	protein
Mixed Type:	335	28g	17g	11g
Carb Type:	298	18g	26g	13g
Protein Type:	382	31g	20g	12g

Cooking Tips

PT: Select spinach as the additional greens, increasing to 4 cups. Use only ½ head broccoli.

CT: Reduce coconut oil to 2 tsp. Increase greens to 3 cups. Reduce coconut milk to 1 cup.

Notes and Suggestions

This blended soup can be made into a whole meal for CT by adding a mixed green or vegetable salad, plus a little protein, perhaps nonfat cottage cheese flecked with chopped chives. PT's will need to serve this with meat or poultry, such as Crunchy Chicken Salad / Casserole or Roasted Tomatillo Turkey Salad. It could also be nice served with broiled lamb chops and Mashed Potatoes.

1 in large soup pan, melt coconut oil and sauté green onions and garlic for 1–2 minutes, until translucent.

2 add chopped broccoli and stir. Cook over medium heat, stirring, until broccoli turns bright green.

3 add basil and additional chopped greens. Cover and steam-sauté for 3–4 more minutes.

4 transfer vegetables into food processor or blender. If using blender, process in two batches. Add a little liquid and process until vegetables start to be smooth.

5 add remaining liquids, salt and hot pepper sauce. Process on high until smooth. Taste. Reheat gently, if necessary, to bring back up to temperature. This is usually not necessary. Serve.

Serves 4. Preparation time: 15 minutes.

Creamy Avocado Soup

This rich and creamy, very quick avocado dream can be served either as a soup or a sauce.

4	med ripe avocados, peeled and pitted
1	clove garlic
3	cups clean, filtered water
1/2	cup fresh lemon juice
1	Tbsp Spike vegetable seasoning or kelp seaweed
1/4	cup fresh parsley

1 using a blender or food processor, process avocados, garlic, water and lemon juice until smooth.

2 add vegetable seasoning and parsley. Blend 1 minute. Serve as refreshing cold, raw soup or sauce.

Serves 4. Preparation time: 5 minutes.

Nutrition Facts

	calories	total fat	carbs	protein
Mixed Type:	299	27g	18g	4g
Carb Type:	150	11g	13g	4g
Protein Type:	379	32g	22g	7g

Cooking Tips

PT: Blend 1/3 cup raw cashew or tahini sesame butter with 1/2 cup of the water until smooth. Add remaining ingredients, cover, and blend. Adjust thickness with more water, if necessary.

CT: Substitute 2 cups fresh, steamed asparagus cuts for 2 of the avocados.

Notes and Suggestions

This soup is best for PT with nut butter as added protein. CT can still get the benefit of the avocado's beneficial fatty acids by substituting steamed asparagus for half of the avocado. To make this into a meal, serve it with your appropriate variation of a lower fat protein and vegetable dish such as Ostrich Stir-Fry for CT. Or with Beef Fajitas for PT. If you find that this soup is too rich, try increasing the proportion of asparagus.

Curried Peanut Soup

If your family likes peanut butter, they're probably going to like this creamy, peanutty soup. Make it spicy or mild, according to taste.

1	Tbsp raw or organic butter
2	med garlic cloves, minced
1	cup chopped onion
1	1" slice ginger root, chopped
1	tsp sea or celtic sea salt
1½	Tbsp curry powder
½	tsp ground cumin seed
½	tsp allspice
2	cups tiny cauliflowerettes
2	cups bok choy or chard, leaf and stem, chopped
2	cups vegetable or chicken stock
½	cup natural peanut butter
1	Tbsp currants, finely minced
¼	tsp plus cayenne or red pepper
1½	cups buttermilk, almond or cashew milk

Nutrition Facts

	calories	total fat	carbs	protein
Mixed Type:	293	19g	21g	14g
Carb Type:	267	16g	23g	11g
protein Type:	372	27g	21g	16g

Cooking Tips

PT: Use almond or cashew milk (page 188).

CT: Substitute reduced fat buttermilk for nut milk to reduce calories. Serve 6 instead of 5.

Notes and Suggestions

This unusual, creamy soup would be excellent served with a venison or beef stew meal for a PT or MX. While CT's should minimize nuts, this soup could be served once in a while with Ostrich Stir-Fry or combined with an extra large portion of Northwoods Broccoli Salad or Rainbow Cabbage Salad for a satisfying meal.

1 in a large sauce or soup pan over medium heat, melt butter. Add garlic, onions, and ginger root, and sauté, stirring frequently, until onions turn translucent.

2 add sea salt, curry, cumin and allspice. Simmer for less than a minute. Add cauliflower and greens, cooking for 3–5 minutes.

3 stir about ¾ cup of stock gradually into peanut butter until smooth. Add remaining stock to vegetables. Stir in diluted peanut butter and heat for 3–5 minutes or until heated through.

4 stir in remaining ingredients and bring back up to temperature. Ladle into serving bowls.

Serves 5. Preparation time: 15 minutes.

Fast French Onion Soup

You'll be surprised at how delicious this fast version of French Onion Soup can be, using high quality ingredients, of course.

2	Tbsp coconut oil, raw or organic butter
3	cloves garlic, minced
3	medium onions, peeled and sliced into rings
1	lb button mushrooms, brushed and sliced
1	Tbsp dried thyme leaves
2	tsp dried marjoram leaves
¼	cup wheat-free tamari soy sauce
2	quarts clean, filtered water, vegetable or free-range chicken stock

1 in a large skillet over medium heat, melt oil. Add garlic and onions, and cook for a few minutes until translucent. Add mushrooms and cook, stirring frequently, until mushrooms are tender, 2 to 3 more minutes. For more flavor, if you have time, sauté onions until they start to caramelize.

2 stir in thyme and marjoram leaves, 1 Tbsp wheat-free tamari. Sauté a few seconds more to let flavors develop.

3 add water and bring soup back up to the boiling point. Reduce heat and simmer 5 more minutes. Add remaining tamari. Serve.

Serves 4. Preparation time: 15 minutes.

Nutrition Facts

	calories	total fat	carbs	protein
Mixed Type:	314	13g	33g	19g
Carb Type:	235	7g	35g	9g
Protein Type:	348	16g	30g	21g

Cooking Tips

PT: Can use chicken stock instead of vegetable stock. Use 2 medium onions. Serve with 2 Tbsp grated Parmesan cheese and 2 Tbsp Savory Sunny Seed Mix (page 215), or both, if desired.

CT: Use vegetable stock. Omit mushrooms.

Notes and Suggestions

Making traditional French onion soup is usually a laborious process of slowly sautéing the onions until caramelized and brown, then thickening and simmering for a long time. This fast version, using high-quality, wheat-free tamari soy sauce, produces an amazingly good soup. Regular commercial soy sauce will not produce the flavor this dish depends upon, in lieu of the traditionally long cooking time. This soup could become a meal with the addition of grated cheese such as Parmesan or Swiss, Savory Sunny Seed Mix and a hearty mixed green or spinach salad with cooked, leftover chicken to satisfy a PT. For a CT meal, sprinkle with either 1 tsp Parmesan cheese or Sunny Seed Gomasio (page 215), and serve with a mixed green salad, or pair with an Egg Salad and Artichoke Roll-Up.

Gazpacho

The quintessential cold summer soup, popular in Spain. Refreshing on a hot night, but even nicer, it's quick, healthy and raw. And there's no need to go near the stove.

Nutrition Facts

	calories	total fat	carbs	protein
Mixed Type:	197	10g	25g	7g
Carb Type:	167	6g	25g	7g

Cooking Tips

PT: Not your best combination of vegetables.

CT: Reduce olive oil to 1 Tbsp.

Notes and Suggestions

This is an ideal CT recipe—light, refreshing, low in fat and protein, with lots of acceptable raw vegetables for your type. You're lucky, it's one of the best cooling summer soups. Serve it with a fresh green salad and chicken for a quick and cooling summer supper.

6	med tomatoes, quartered
2	large cucumbers, chopped
1	small red onion
1	med zucchini, chopped
3	med garlic cloves, smashed
1	med green bell pepper
3/4	cup chopped fresh herbs: parsley, basil, chives
2	Tbsp lemon juice or 1 Tbsp red wine vinegar
2	Tbsp extra virgin olive oil
1	tsp sea salt or Spike vegetable seasoning
1/2	tsp cayenne pepper or 1 jalapeño, seeded
1	tsp ground cumin seed
2	cups vegetable stock or tomato juice

1 in food processor, combine tomatoes, cucumbers, onion, zucchini, garlic, and green pepper and process on high until coarsely chopped.

2 add herbs, lemon juice, oil, salt, cayenne or jalapeño, and cumin. Process a few more bursts. Blend in stock or tomato juice.

3 transfer to large bowl or glass container. Refrigerate at least 1 hour before serving.

Serves 4. Preparation time: 10 minutes.

Greek Egg-Lemon Soup

This classic Greek soup is called Avgolemono (that's why we called it Egg-Lemon). It's velvety smooth with a sharp, lemony tang...steamy perfection on a cool fall evening.

2	32 oz free-range chicken stock
1	Tbsp raw or organic butter
2	tsp onion powder
½	tsp sea or celtic sea salt
¾	cup fresh lemon juice
1	tsp dried oregano leaves
3	large eggs
½	cup fresh parsley, finely chopped

1 in large saucepan, heat chicken broth and butter over medium. Reduce heat.

2 add onion powder, salt, lemon juice, and oregano. Stir to blend well.

3 break eggs into small bowl. Whisk with a wire whip until blended, but not frothy.

4 while soup simmers, ladle out about ⅔ cup hot broth and stir into beaten eggs to temper or raise temperature of eggs.

5 gently pour egg-broth mixture slowly back into soup in saucepan, whisking constantly. DO NOT BOIL. Remove from heat, ladle into bowls and sprinkle with chopped parsley.

Serves 4. Preparation time: 10 minutes.

Nutrition Facts

	calories	total fat	carbs	protein
Mixed Type:	134	7g	8g	12g
Carb Type:	134	7g	8g	12g
Protein Type:	177	11g	8g	13g

Cooking Tips

PT: Use 2 Tbsp butter. Use 4 eggs.

CT: Follow as is.

Notes and Suggestions

This traditional soup is a light accompaniment to salads, Grilled Herbed Salmon or chicken or lamb for a PT. Add a vegetable like Lemon Pepper Green Beans and enjoy a satisfying meal. CT could make a balanced menu combining a larger, double portion with a Middle Eastern Salad and a little extra feta or lowfat farmer cheese.

Lickety Split Chicken Soup

A fast solution for a busy day when dinner's the last thing on your list.

1	Tbsp organic butter or coconut oil
1	med onion, diced
3	stalks celery, chopped
1	cup baby carrots, sliced in half
2	cups diced cabbage
2	cups frozen organic green bean cuts
6	cups free-range chicken broth
2	tsp thyme leaves
1	tsp sea salt or Spike vegetable seasoning
2	cups clean, filtered water
1½	lb free-range chicken, roasted
1	Tbsp fresh or dried chopped parsley

Nutrition Facts

	calories	total fat	carbs	protein
Mixed Type:	230	8g	18g	24g
Carb Type:	202	3g	15g	29g
Protein Type:	241	10g	20g	19g

Cooking Tips

PT: This has a lot of vegetables recommended for your type, so it's a good recipe for you. Increase butter to 2 Tbsp, celery to 5 stalks. Choose 2 lb predominantly dark leftover chicken.

CT: Follow the recipe as is or you can substitute chopped broccoli, diced turnips, diced zucchini, or peppers. Use 2 cups chicken breast.

Notes and Suggestions

This can be a meal in itself for all types. Just watch proportions and optimum foods. For example, PT's will need to add the most chicken (dark), CT's the least (white), and MX somewhere in between (both dark and white meat). The exact amounts that are right for you will depend upon your individual system. This is something you will begin to learn through your own experience, trial and error testing. So, as with any recipe, start with the guidelines given, then adjust amounts and specific foods to your own particular needs, as you fine-tune your body awareness.

1 place large heavy soup kettle on medium high heat. Add butter and onion, celery, carrots, and cabbage. Stir, cooking until vegetables start to give off steam. Add green beans and pour over ½ cup of the chicken broth. Cover and steam 4–5 minutes.

2 remove cover, add remaining chicken stock, thyme leaves, salt, and water. Cover and bring back up to a boil. Continue cooking for 4–5 minutes.

3 while stock is simmering, cut up roast chicken into ½" pieces. Add chicken and parsley to soup. Heat 3–4 minutes more until heated through. Serve immediately.

Serves 4. Preparation time: 15 minutes.

Maestro's Minestrone

This classic Italian supper soup is a rainbow of garden colors and flavors in a bowl.

1	Tbsp extra virgin olive oil
4	med garlic cloves, smashed
1	med red onion, chopped
1	med carrot, chopped
3	stalks celery, chopped
1	med zucchini, quarter sliced
1	Tbsp Italian seasoning
1	tsp celery salt
½	tsp freshly ground black pepper
1	quart vegetable or free-range chicken stock
2	med tomatoes, seeded and chopped
1	cup green cabbage, shredded
½	cup Basil Pesto (page 239)

1 in large kettle or soup pot heated over medium, sauté smashed garlic and onion in olive oil until translucent, about 2 minutes.

2 add chopped carrot, celery, and zucchini, and stir-sauté, stirring frequently, for 5 minutes.

3 add Italian seasoning, chopped tomatoes, celery salt, black pepper, and stock. Bring to a boil. Reduce heat slightly and simmer, covered, for about 6–7 minutes. Add cabbage.

4 taste and adjust seasoning. Ladle into soup bowls and top with 1 Tbsp Basil Pesto per serving.

5 serve immediately when you're in a hurry. But remember that soup develops more flavor, if allowed to simmer slowly for awhile.

Serves 4. Preparation time: 20 minutes.

Nutrition Facts

	calories	total fat	carbs	protein
Mixed Type:	319	21g	23g	13g
Carb Type:	192	9g	21g	9g
Protein Type:	322	21g	23g	14g

Cooking Tips

PT: Could increase celery to 4 stalks, add 2 cups chopped spinach, omitting cabbage.

CT: Reduce Pesto to 1 tsp per serving.

Notes and Suggestions

CT's could add ⅔ cup cooked navy or white beans and ½ cup cooked, leftover chicken to make this an authentic meal in a bowl. For PT's, add leftover meatballs, meatloaf or diced beef or bison. This soup would also be delicious served with a mixed green salad and Parmesan Crisps.

Miso Soup with Watercress

A speedy, but satisfying vegetarian soup with a hearty meaty-like flavor, thanks to the Oriental staple, miso, a fermented soybean paste.

10	oz extra firm tofu, cut into 1/2" cubes
1	32 oz container vegetable broth Or free-range chicken broth
2	cups clean, filtered water
1/4	cup white, dark brown or red miso paste
1/2	cup water chestnuts
1	bunch fresh watercress, cut in 1/2" pieces
1	tsp roasted sesame oil

1 in saucepan, combine tofu cubes with broth. Dissolve miso in 1/2 cup water and add with remaining water and water chestnuts to saucepan.

2 heat lightly over medium low until just heated through. Add watercress pieces and roasted sesame oil.

3 ladle into soup bowls and serve immediately.

Serves 4. Preparation time: 10 minutes.

Nutrition Facts

	calories	*total fat*	*carbs*	*protein*
Mixed Type:	286	10g	35g	16g
Carb Type:	221	7g	30g	10g
Protein Type:	321	13g	37g	18g

Cooking Tips

PT: Increase tofu to 12 oz. Increase sesame oil to 2 tsp.

CT: Reduce tofu to 5 oz. Increase water chestnuts to 3/4 cup.

Notes and Suggestions

The best soyfoods to eat are fermented foods like miso, natto and tempeh, which do not contain the enzyme inhibitors in soybeans. Other soy products, such as tofu, should only be used very occasionally.

Mushroom Cream Soup

This creamy mushroom soup is almost as fast as the commercial kind to pre-pare and, we're sure you'll agree, MUCH better tasting.

2	Tbsp raw or organic butter
2	cloves garlic, minced
3	green onions, sliced
1½	lb fresh button mushrooms, chopped
2	tsp dried thyme leaves
2	tsp dried marjoram leaves
2	Tbsp tamari soy sauce
2	Tbsp arrowroot
6	cups clean, filtered water
½	cup raw or organic half and half cream or lite coconut milk

1 in a large skillet heat butter over medium high heat. Add garlic and onions. Cook for 1 minute.

2 add mushrooms, thyme, and marjoram leaves, cook about 5 minutes, until mushrooms are tender. Add tamari. Sauté a few seconds more.

3 dissolve arrowroot in 1 cup of the water. Add this with remaining water and bring soup back up to the boiling point. Continue cooking, stirring frequently, 5–6 minutes until soup thickens.

4 remove from heat. Add half and half or coconut milk. Pour soup into blender container, cover and process on high until smooth and creamy. Serve.

Serves 4. Preparation time: 15 minutes.

Nutrition Facts

	calories	total fat	carbs	protein
Mixed Type:	156	10g	13g	8g
Carb Type:	128	9g	11g	5g
Protein Type:	182	11g	15g	10g

Cooking Tips

PT: Increase butter to 2 Tbsp. Double the mushrooms. Increase half and half to ⅔ cup.

CT: While mushrooms are not your top-of-the-list vegetable, you can enjoy this soup occasionally. See how you feel using ½ cup lite coconut milk instead of half and half.

Notes and Suggestions

To make this into a complete meal for MX or PT, it could be served with Steaming Chicken with Vegetables or a vegetable-meat combination like Broccoli-in-a-Hurry Curry Dressing and Horseradish Buffalo Burgers. CT could also combine the soup with Steaming Chicken and Vegetables for a healthy and satisfying meal.

Oriental Hot & Sour Mushroom Egg Drop

This amalgam of hot and sour, Chinese mushroom, and egg drop soup combines the flavors and textures of all three.

1	Tbsp roasted sesame oil
3	slices fresh ginger root
4	med green onions, sliced
1/2	lb shiitake mushrooms, sliced
2	8 oz. cans bamboo shoots, drained
2/3	cup water chestnuts, drained and thinly sliced
3	Tbsp wheat-free tamari soy sauce
2	32 oz free-range chicken broth
4	cups Chinese cabbage, shredded
2	cups snow pea pods, in 1" diagonal cuts
2	Tbsp rice wine vinegar
3	med eggs, beaten

Nutrition Facts

	calories	total fat	carbs	protein
Mixed Type:	225	8g	25g	18g
Carb Type:	198	5g	26g	16g
Protein Type:	253	8g	29g	19g

Cooking Tips

PT: Increase mushrooms to 1 lb. Add 1 more egg.

CT: Decrease oil to 2 tsp.

Notes and Suggestions

This dish has the components of a main meal in itself, but decrease serving size to 2. PT will want to add dark meat chicken, sliced beef, meat balls or even fish, as will MX, who should serve a smaller amount. CT: This will likely work for you as it stands, with a larger portion.

1 heat large saucepan or skillet over medium high heat. Add sesame oil and ginger slices and sauté for several minutes.

2 add white parts of onions, mushrooms, bamboo shoots, and water chestnuts, and sauté over medium heat, stirring frequently, for 5 minutes.

3 add tamari soy sauce and stock. Simmer, covered for about 8–10 minutes.

4 add Chinese cabbage, snow peas, and vinegar about 5–6 minutes before ready to serve. Get serving bowls or tureen ready.

5 heat the soup to a gentle boil. Stir soup in a circular direction with a knife or chopstick, drizzling the beaten egg in a thin steady stream. Remove from heat. Serve with scallion top garnish.

Serves 4. Preparation time: 20 minutes.

Quick Miso Cup

A quick pick-me-up to satisfy hunger between meals.

1½   **cups clean, filtered water**
1   **Tbsp white, brown or dark red miso paste**
½   **green onion, sliced**

1 heat water. Place miso in soup cup or small bowl. Add hot water gradually and stir to dissolve.

2 sprinkle with green onion slices. Serve immediately.

Serves 1. Preparation time: 5 minutes.

Nutrition Facts

calories	total fat	carbs	protein
38	1g	5g	2g

Cooking Tips

Varying this soup for each type will depend upon the foods eaten with it. PT: You can try eating this with celery stuffed with Sesame Miso Spread or chicken salad as a snack.

CT: Enjoy this cup-o'-soup with sprouts or a small mixed green salad, which should be satisfying for you as a pick-me-up.

Notes and Suggestions

Miso is an ancient Chinese, salty, soybean paste, fermented to be more digestible and acceptable as a soyfood. It can be added as a flavoring and protein enhancer to soups, sauces, dips and spreads, or simply diluted in hot water for a quick snack like this soup. Miso is actually a live food, so do not boil. Add it at the end to any hot recipe.

Roasted Tomatillo Turkey Soup

A chameleon recipe that transforms a tasty south-of-the-border salad into a hearty, cold weather soup.

1   **Recipe Roasted Tomatillo Turkey Salad (page 163)**

1   **quart free-range chicken broth**

¼   **cup Green Olive Tomatillo Salsa for garnish (page 243)**

1 bring chicken broth to a boil.

2 add hot chicken broth to prepared salad in a bowl or saucepan.

3 ready to serve! Hot chicken broth warms the ingredients. No further heating really required.

Serves 4. Preparation time: 5 minutes.

Nutrition Facts

	calories	*total fat*	*carbs*	*protein*
Mixed Type:	338	17g	15g	31g
Carb Type:	274	13g	9g	221g
Protein Type:	402	27g	13g	40g

Cooking Tips

PT: OK as is. Add ⅓ cup Green Olive Tomatillo Salsa on top, if desired, for garnish

CT: Use your version of Roasted Tomatillo Turkey Salad or reduce amount of turkey salad, made with breast meat, to 2 cups. Reduce Green Olive Salsa garnish to 2 Tbsp. Add or serve with 1 cup clover or mixed sprouts per serving.

Notes and Suggestions

Use your version of Roasted Tomatillo Salad to make this almost instant soup. Once again, this quick, convertible recipe is one to vary with accompaniments. PT's should be fine with the recipe as it is, but may want to serve it with an avocado and sprout Roll-Up. CT's could complement the soup with salad and/or sprouts. Regardless of what the recipe suggests, it's up to you to find the balance of ingredients that works best for you.

THE RECIPES: Main Dishes

The recipes here, as well as the recipes throughout the entire cookbook, can actually be enjoyed for any meal, anytime. You can have steak and vegetables for breakfast, as well as lunch or dinner. In smaller quantities, you can even have them as a snack. That's because the overriding emphasis of the Total Health Program is to keep your blood sugar stable by consuming a balance of nutrients as close to your ideal ratio of fats, carbohydrates and protein as possible, each and every time you eat.

This section is divided into five areas: 1) Beef; 2) Bison, Ostrich and Other Meats; 3) Free-Range Poultry—Chicken and Turkey; 4) No-Meat Main Dishes; and 5) Safe Salmon Dishes.

Please pay attention to the very clear, specific and repeated references to acceptable protein sources. As stated in Part One, the quality or form of the protein you eat is extremely important —as important as the actual amount you consume on a daily basis. That is why here and throughout this book you will find certain specific brands and types of meats, fish, poultry and dairy recommended, with information about where you can find them. Eating the best forms of foods as well as the right quantities will make all the difference in your health.

Beef 'n Beer Stew

Good old fashioned beef stew done in a crockpot can be a warm welcome home at the end of a long, cold day.

2	Tbsp coconut oil
1	lb beef round or stew meat, cut into 1" cubes
1	tsp salt
½	tsp freshly ground black pepper
¾	cup chopped onion
5	med garlic cloves, pressed
1	bay leaf
1	Tbsp thyme leaves
2	Tbsp tomato paste
2	Tbsp Worcestershire sauce
¾	cup baby carrots
4	stalks celery, cut into 2" ribs
2	med kohlrabi, peeled, sliced and quartered
1	lb fresh mushrooms, cut in half
3	cups clean, filtered water
3	cups natural beef stock
1	12 oz bottle stout or other dark beer
½	cup chopped parsley

Nutrition Facts

	calories	total fat	carbs	protein
Mixed Type:	349	12g	23g	35g
Carb Type:	174	4g	24g	9g
Protein Type:	384	13g	21g	43g

Cooking Tips

PT: Increase beef to 1¼ lb. Increase mushrooms to 1½ lb and celery to 5 stalks.

CT: Reduce coconut oil to 1 Tbsp. Use ostrich chuck or stew meat and reduce to 12 oz for the recipe. Could increase kohlrabi to 3.

Notes and Suggestions

Beef stew—or any meat stew—is a classic meat and vegetable combination, a stand-alone meal in itself. One of the nice things about this type of dish is that it can be simmering all day in a crockpot, ready to eat when you walk in the door.

1 heat large heavy kettle or stockpot to medium high or crockpot to high heat. While heating, sprinkle beef with salt and pepper. Add oil and sauté beef, stirring frequently, for 7–9 minutes until browned. Remove beef pieces and hold.

2 add onions, garlic, bay leaves, and thyme to pan and sauté until translucent. Stir in tomato paste, Worcestershire sauce.

3 add carrots, celery, kohlrabi, and mushrooms. Stir to coat and sauté a few minutes. Add browned beef, water, stock, and beer.

4 reduce to low and simmer, covered, for several hours, until beef is tender. Ladle into bowls and serve, sprinkled with chopped parsley.

Serves 4. Preparation time: 15 minutes.

Beef Fajitas

Fajitas, a popular Mexican entrée these days, can be enjoyed on this eating plan by selecting the optimum meats and vegetables for each type.

1	Tbsp coconut oil
1	med red onion, sliced
1½	cups green bell pepper strips
1½	cups yellow bell pepper strips
3	stalks celery, cut on diagonal
2	med zucchini, cut into ½" diagonal slices
2	Tbsp fajita seasoning made with:
	2 Tbsp chili powder, 1 Tbsp cumin, 1 tsp each
	oregano and garlic powder
1	lb grass-fed beef steak, sliced crossgrain
½	cup salsa
½	cup Chunky Mockamole (page 241)
	Parmesan Crisps (optional, page 218)

1 heat a large skillet over medium high heat. Add coconut oil and sauté onions, peppers, celery, zucchini, and fajita seasoning until onions are translucent. Remove vegetables and hold.

2 add beef slices and sauté until pink is gone. Add reserved vegetables and bring back up to temperature.

3 serve with salsa or Green Olive Tomatillo Salsa and Chunky Mockamole, along with 2 Parmesan Crisps, recipes you can find in the Condiments & Extra's and Quick Snacks chapters.

Serves 4. Preparation time: 10 minutes.

Nutrition Facts

	calories	total fat	carbs	protein
Mixed Type:	362	18g	18g	33g
Carb Type:	280	8g	25g	30g
Protein Type:	395	21g	11g	40g

Cooking Tips

PT: Increase beef to 1¼ lb. Use ½ red onion in preparation. Increase celery to 6 stalks, reduce peppers to 1½ cups total.

CT: Use ostrich steak or strips, and reduce meat to 12 oz. Increase salsa to ⅔ cup and reduce Chunky Mockamole to 1 Tbsp per serving.

Notes and Suggestions

A natural meal-in-one recipe, fajitas can be adjusted to fit your type by varying the vegetables, meat and condiments. PT and MX might want to serve these with Parmesan Crisps. CT, with less protein and more carbohydrate requirements, could add a tossed salad with Basic Herb Vinaigrette (page 241) for a balanced menu.

Beef Pot Roast with Sauerkraut

Lower fat, tougher cuts of meat become flavorful and very tender when slow-simmered with sauerkraut.

3$\frac{1}{2}$	lb grass-fed beef rump roast, bottom round or brisket
	salt and pepper to taste
1	Tbsp coconut oil
$\frac{1}{2}$	cup chopped onions
1	tsp thyme leaves
2	lb sauerkraut
2	small apples, quartered
2	bay leaves OR
1	Tbsp mixed pickling spices (bay leaves, mustard seed, ginger, cinnamon, red and black pepper, caraway seeds, cloves, mace, allspice, cardamom)
2	cups boiling water or natural beef stock
4	med kohlrabi, peeled and quartered
2	small turnips
4	stalks celery
4	med carrots, cut in thirds

Nutrition Facts

	calories	total fat	carbs	protein
Mixed Type:	375	11g	20g	36g
Carb Type:	302	7g	20g	32g
Protein Type:	416	9g	23g	38g

Cooking Tips

PT: Serve slightly larger portions to 7 instead of 8.

CT: Beef is not the best meat for your type. Try this slow-simmered recipe with sauerkraut and vegetables, substituting 2 lb ostrich "stew meat" or chicken breast. Reduce cook time to under 1 hour.

Notes and Suggestions

This one-dish-meal could be prepared in a crockpot, yielding plenty of leftovers for a PT or MX. The preplanning required is the primary effort.

1 season the meat with salt and pepper. In crockpot or large Dutch oven or heavy pot over medium high, melt coconut oil. Brown the beef on both sides with the onions. Add thyme leaves.

2 cover with sauerkraut and apple quarters, bay leaves or pickling spices. Add 2 cups boiling water or stock. Cover and simmer several hours or until tender.

3 for maximum nutrition, steam vegetables in steamer basket over boiling water just before ready to serve. To maximize flavor and time, vegetables can be added with the sauerkraut and simmered as the meat tenderizes.

Serves 8. Preparation time: 15 minutes.

Herb-Seasoned Steak Broil

This is a fast and tasty, center-of-the-plate dinner option, ready in a few short minutes.

1	lb grass-fed top sirloin steak
2	tsp coconut oil
2	Tbsp Dijon mustard
2	tsp grated or prepared horseradish
2	tsp dried thyme leaves
1	tsp ground celery seed
1	tsp onion powder
1	tsp coarse sea or celtic salt
1/2	tsp freshly ground black pepper

1 take steak out of refrigerator at least 1/2 hour before serving. Preheat oven to Broil. Set oven rack 6" from broiler unit.

2 rub both sides of steak with coconut oil. Mix Dijon mustard and horseradish together. Spread evenly over both sides of meat. Place meat on lightly greased broiler pan.

3 in small cup, mix thyme leaves, ground celery seed, onion powder, coarse salt and ground pepper. Divide mixture, sprinkling half on each side of meat.

4 broil steak 3-4 minutes on each side, or until browned on top. Remove to serving platter, let rest 1 minute. Slice and serve.

Serves 5. Preparation time: 10 minutes.

Nutrition Facts

	calories	total fat	carbs	protein
Mixed Type:	254	14g	2g	28g
Carb Type:	176	6g	2g	27g
Protein Type:	315	18g	2g	35g

Cooking Tips

PT: This is a PT kind of entrée. Serve 4.

CT: Beef is not a recommended meat for CT, so skip this or use the recipe, substituting ostrich strip steaks and reducing oil to 2 tsp.

Notes and Suggestions

PT's, with the highest protein requirements, will still need to add vegetables and/or a salad to make this a balanced meal. A Caesar-type salad made with more than half spinach or a Middle Eastern Salad could serve the purpose.

Quick Beef Steaks with Mushrooms and Wine

Using grass-fed beef cube steaks can shorten cooking time and calories. For more flavor, marinate ahead.

4	large grass-fed beef cube steaks
1/2	cup red wine
8	oz fresh mushrooms, quartered
2	med garlic cloves, minced
2	Tbsp finely chopped parsley
2	Tbsp raw or organic butter

1 several hours before serving, if possible, place cube steaks in quart-size plastic bag, then set in a bowl to help bag stand up. Add wine, mushrooms, minced garlic and parsley. Let marinate a minimum of half an hour for flavor, or for more tender cuts, up to, but no more than, 24 hours.

2 heat large skillet over medium high heat. Melt butter. Place steaks, two at a time, in hot pan. Braise for 2 minutes on a side. Remove to serving platter or shallow casserole.

3 pour reserved marinade into pan and bring back up to boil. Cook for a couple of minutes, then pour over steaks. Remove to platter and serve immediately.

4 if you don't have time, simply heat marinade ingredients together in a small pan for 2–3 minutes, while searing steaks in butter, as directed. Remove from pan.

5 add marinade and deglaze or scrape up any of the flavorful browned bits from cooking the meat on the bottom of the pan. Pour over steaks. No tenderizing benefit this way, and flavor won't be as intense, but it will still be good.

Serves 4. Preparation time: 10 minutes.

Nutrition Facts

	calories	total fat	carbs	protein
Mixed Type:	279	11g	3g	35g
Carb Type:	173	7g	3g	25g
Protein Type:	345	15g	5g	47g

Cooking Tips

PT: Increase mushrooms to 1–12 oz package or even 1 lb, if you like them. Stir in 2 Tbsp sour cream just before serving.

CT: Use 12 oz ostrich strip steaks for this recipe. Decrease butter to 1 Tbsp.

Notes and Suggestions

You could serve this quick meal with Brussels Sprouts Trio or a simple steamed broccoli or a salad. CT's might want to serve both a vegetable and salad with a smaller portion of meat.

Steak Tartare

The classic raw gourmet presentation, Steak Tartare originates with the nomadic Tartars, who were so busy, with no time to cook, they pulverized their meat under their saddles. You can use a food processor.

1	lb grass-fed beef tenderloin or sirloin steak
1	Tbsp capers
2	tsp Dijon mustard
2	tsp Worcestershire sauce
2	Tbsp chopped curly parsley
1	tsp sea salt, celtic gray salt, or kosher salt
4–5	grinds fresh black pepper
8	leaves romaine or butter lettuce
4	raw egg yolks
½	small red onion, sliced into rings

1 cut up meat into 4–5 chunks. Process in food processor until finely chopped.

2 combine ground steak, most of the capers, Dijon mustard, Worcestershire sauce, chopped parsley, salt and pepper. Shape into patties and let rest for a few minutes to allow flavors to blend.

3 line serving plates with romaine or butter lettuce. The classic presentation consists of a raw ground steak patty with a spoon-sized hollow for a perfect raw egg yolk, topped with raw onion rings and sprinkled with a few more capers.

Serves 4. Preparation time: 10 minutes.

Nutrition Facts

	calories	total fat	carbs	protein
Mixed Type:	254	14g	3g	28g
Carb Type:	205	12g	3g	20g
Protein Type:	273	15g	2g	31g

Cooking Tips

PT: Add 1 Tbsp Dijon Remoulade Sauce (page 238) per serving, if desired.

CT: This is just not your kind of dish, unless you use 12 oz ground ostrich filet, increase parsley to ⅓ cup, and serve 3 raw "meat balls" per serving, with a salad or vegetable crudité (cut-up raw vegetables.)

Notes and Suggestions

If you're not used to the raw egg yolks, you can combine them with the rest of the ingredients in Step 2. If the raw meat doesn't appeal to you, you can broil it like a burger. To balance this as a meal, PT could serve it with Fast French Onion Soup and a Caesar Salad. CT could opt for the soup and a simple green salad or a platter of fresh vegetables like Kohlrabi and Side Kickers.

Sukiyaki with Beef

The traditional Japanese "Friendship" Dish, this classic beef and vegetable one dish meal is a fast and easy Sunday or any night supper for family or guests.

2	large garlic cloves, minced
1/4	cup tamari soy sauce
1 1/2	Tbsp Worcestershire sauce
2	Tbsp Mirin, rice wine vinegar
1 1/2	lb grass-fed beef flank or strip steak
1	Tbsp coconut oil
2	large stalks celery, cut on diagonal (about 2 cups)
1 1/2	med yellow onions, crescent-sliced (about 2 cups)
1/8	head shredded green cabbage (about 2 cups)
4	cups shredded Swiss chard, Bok choy or Chinese cabbage
2	cups sliced mushrooms
4	med scallions or green onions, cut diagonally into thirds
1	can bamboo shoots (about 1 cup) plus liquid
1	can water chestnuts (about 1 cup) plus liquid
1 3/4	cups natural beef or free-range chicken stock
2	Tbsp arrowroot flour (page 252)
6	cups Zucchetti Pasta (page 234) or Spaghetti Squash (page 107)

Nutrition Facts

	calories	total fat	carbs	protein
Mixed Type:	392	18g	24g	37g
Carb Type:	140	4g	24g	8g
Protein Type:	419	20g	23g	41g

Cooking Tips

PT: Can increase beef to 2 lb and serve 7 with this recipe.

CT: Beef is not one of your best recommended meats, but you could make this recipe with ostrich strip steaks or chicken breast.

Serves 6. Preparation time: 20 minutes.

1 mix minced garlic, soy sauce, Worcestershire sauce, and rice wine vinegar in medium mixing bowl or covered container.

2 cut steak across the grain into thin slices or strips with a sharp knife. This is easier to do if the meat is partially frozen. Add meat strips to marinade in bowl and stir to coat beef. If using flank steak, marinate several hours to help tenderize. If using more tender cuts of steak, long marinating is not required.

3 have all vegetables cut up and close at hand. When ready to cook, drain meat from marinade and reserve both. Heat spun steel wok or large, heavy frying pan over high. Melt coconut oil, add drained beef.

4 sauté, stirring constantly, for about 1 minute, till meat loses some pinkness. If using wok, pull meat up the sides of wok, or remove from skillet and keep warm. Add stock and juices from bamboo shoots and water chestnuts to marinade in bowl. Add celery and onions to wok, stirring for 1–2 minutes. Pour 1/4 cup stock over to create steam. Add shredded cabbage, chard and stir-fry until these veggies start to wilt. Pour over 1/4 cup more stock to create steam and shorten veggie cooking time.

5 reduce heat to medium or medium low. Add mushrooms, scallions, bamboo shoots, water chestnuts and beef slices to wok. Stir to mix.

6 drain off liquid from bottom of wok into marinade/stock mixture. Blend in 2 Tbsp arrowroot flour with wire whisk. Pour back into wok and stir until thickened. Pour over vegetables and beef. Serve as is, or over Zucchetti or steamed spaghetti squash.

Buffalo Chili

This might be a good recipe for trying bison meat, to discover that it tastes a lot like beef, only better.

1	Tbsp coconut oil
1/2	cup chopped onions
2	med garlic cloves, minced
1 1/2	cups chopped celery
1	cup chopped green pepper
1 1/2	lb ground bison or buffalo meat (page 251)
2	tsp thyme leaves
2	tsp chili powder
2	tsp ground cumin
1	tsp sea salt
1	8 oz can tomatoes
1	12 oz jar prepared salsa

1 in large skillet or crockpot on medium to high, melt oil and sauté onions, garlic, celery, and pepper until onion is translucent, 3–4 minutes.

2 add ground meat, thyme, chili powder and cumin, and cook, stirring frequently, for 5–6 minutes.

3 pour salt, tomatoes, and salsa into pot. Cover, reduce heat and simmer for a minimum of 1 hour. Crockpot on low can simmer for quite a few hours.

4 serve in bowls or over tiny steamed cauliflowerettes.

Serves 4. Preparation time: 15 minutes.

Nutrition Facts

	calories	total fat	carbs	protein
Mixed Type:	284	7g	19g	38g
Carb Type:	229	6g	36g	12g
Protein Type:	319	10g	14g	43g

Cooking Tips

PT: Use $1^3/4$ lb ground meat. Decrease onion to $1/2$ cup. Increase chopped celery to $2^1/2$ cups.

CT: Reduce coconut oil to 1 Tbsp. Increase onion to 1 cup. Add 1 med green pepper, seeded and chopped. Substitute ground ostrich or turkey breast meat. Use 1–16 oz can tomatoes.

Notes and Suggestions

This is a popular winter favorite that can be made healthier by using bison or buffalo meat and varied for type with appropriate vegetables and meats. Excellent accompaniments are traditional coleslaw, Sunny Rainbow Cabbage Salad, or Northwoods Broccoli Salad.

Herbed Lemony Lamb Chops

Lamb chops with this lemony flavor treatment are delicious, whatever cut you can afford.

4	lamb shoulder chops
1	tsp grated lemon peel (no white) or
½	tsp lemon pepper seasoning
½	tsp dried rosemary, crushed
1	tsp dried oregano
1	tsp dried tarragon
3	Tbsp lemon juice
1	Tbsp tamari soy sauce

Nutrition Facts

	calories	*total fat*	*carbs*	*protein*
Mixed Type:	317	21g	2g	28g
Protein Type:	423	29g	2g	37g

Cooking Tips

Since this is basically a meat recipe, adjust the menu with vegetables and other foods to fit your specific metabolic needs.

PT: Can increase portion size and serve 3–4 with this recipe, instead of 4.

CT: Lamb is not one of your recommended meats. Try making this recipe with chicken breast or fish instead.

Notes and Suggestions

Serve the lamb chops with Greek Egg-Lemon Soup and a healthy portion of Braised Brazilian Greens, or Grecian Spinach for a traditional Mediterranean meal. Or pair them with Grilled Ratatouille Salad or Middle Eastern Salad.

1 heat large skillet over medium high heat. Brown lamb chops on both sides.

2 combine lemon peel, herbs, lemon juice and tamari in small bowl. Pour over chops in pan. Cover and simmer over medium low for 20–25 minutes, or until tender.

3 this could also be used as a seasoning "paste" or pesto for broiling loin lamb chops. Simply reduce lemon juice in herb mixture to 1 Tbsp, making a paste. Spread on loin chops and broil 3–4 minutes per side, depending upon thickness. Do not overcook.

Serves 4. Preparation time: 10 minutes.

Horseradish Buffalo Burgers

Bison or buffalo meat tastes surprisingly like beef and is lower in both calories and fat.

1	**lb ground bison or buffalo meat (page 251)**
2	**Tbsp prepared horseradish**
½	**tsp Spike vegetable seasoning or Mrs. Dash**
3–4	**grinds fresh black pepper**

1 combine ground bison and remaining ingredients. Form into patties.

2 broil in the oven or over a grill, or fry in hot, cast iron skillet over medium high, 3–4 minutes on a side, until browned. DO NOT over-cook. Serve immediately.

Serves 4. Preparation time: 10 minutes.

Nutrition Facts

	calories	*total fat*	*carbs*	*protein*
Mixed Type:	259	18g	1g	21g
Protein Type:	322	23g	1g	27g

Cooking Tips

PT: Can increase meat to 1¹/4 lb.

CT: Not your recommended meat, so prepare this with ground ostrich or turkey, as an alternate.

Notes and Suggestions

This recipe goes nicely with Roasted Asparagus or Green Bean Casserole. If still hungry, try adding a salad or another vegetable. The process of experimentation is what this eating plan is all about.

Oriental Ostrich Salad

You'll find this Asian-inspired beef and sesame salad to be an excellent main entrée prepared with ostrich or grass-fed beef.

1	1b ostrich filet or steak strips (page 253)
3	Tbsp Mirin, rice vinegar
1	1" piece fresh ginger root, grated
3	quarts mesclun or leafy spring greens mix
1	cup coarsely shredded red cabbage
1	cup mung bean sprouts
1/2	cup radish sprouts
4	Tbsp Asian Dressing (page 236)
1	Tbsp toasted sesame seed

Nutrition Facts

	calories	total fat	carbs	protein
Mixed Type:	297	12g	15g	33g
Carb Type:	245	10g	16g	29g
Protein Type:	383	23g	18g	37g

Cooking Tips

PT: Ostrich is a lower fat meat, not as recommended for PT. Substitute 12 oz grass-fed beef or bison filet. Add 1 Tbsp sesame seeds and 2 Tbsp Asian Dressing.

CT: Ostrich is ideal for your type. Use 12 oz ostrich filets, omit or reduce sesame seeds, substituting 1/4 cup sliced waterchestnuts.

Notes and Suggestions

Ostrich is much lower in fat than beef and cooks faster. Do Not Overcook. Remember, meat continues to cook after you take it off the heat.

1 marinate ostrich steak filets in vinegar and grated ginger for 20–30 minutes, up to 2 hours, while preparing other ingredients.

2 grill ostrich steaks over lightly greased grill or ridged grill pan on medium, 1–2 minutes per side, until medium rare. Remove from heat and transfer meat to cutting board to rest 5 minutes. If using filet, slice steak thinly across the grain.

3 meanwhile, prepare serving platter or individual plates with 2–3 cups of the greens, topped with red cabbage shreds, mung bean and radish sprouts.

4 top with grilled ostrich filet strips and drizzle Asian Dressing over top. Sprinkle with sesame seeds.

Serves 4. Preparation time: 15 minutes.

Ostrich Meat Balls with Mushroom Gravy

This relatively quick meatball and mushroom dish is even tastier with ostrich than with beef. Make it faster by skipping the meatball prep and frying the meat quickly with the onions.

Crème Fraîche

1	lb ground ostrich (page 253)
1	tsp dried onion flakes
2	Tbsp finely chopped parsley
2	tsp thyme leaves
1	med whole egg
2	Tbsp coconut oil
1/2	small onion, finely chopped
8	oz mushrooms, sliced
2	Tbsp Beans 'R' Us bean flour, arrowroot or soy flour (page 252)
2	cups clean, filtered water
1	Tbsp tamari soy sauce
1/2	tsp Angoustura Bitters or Worcestershire sauce
1/4	cup Crème Fraîche or sour cream (page 230)

1 combine ground ostrich with onion flakes, parsley, 1 tsp thyme, and egg. Shape into 1" to 1½" meatballs.

2 heat medium skillet over medium high. Melt coconut oil, add onions, add meatballs, 1 tsp of the thyme leaves. Sauté quickly, just until browned on all sides, about 2 minutes. Add mushrooms and remaining thyme leaves, and sauté 1–2 minutes more.

3 add flour and stir to coat, heating for 20–30 seconds. Stir in water and cook, stirring frequently, until mixture is thickened. Remove from heat and stir in soy sauce, bitters and sour cream. Ready to serve.

Serves 4. Preparation time: 15 minutes.

Nutrition Facts

	calories	*total fat*	*carbs*	*protein*
Mixed Type:	342	23g	7g	28g
Carb Type:	270	15g	6g	28g
Protein Type:	428	33g	7g	26g

Cooking Tips

PT: Substitute grass-fed beef or bison, since ostrich is not a recommended meat for you. Increase mushrooms to 12 oz.

CT: Reduce oil to 1 Tbsp and omit sour cream.

Notes and Suggestions

Serve this over Zucchetti Pasta or Mashed Fotatoes for some healthy winter comfort food.

Ostrich Stir-Fry

Ostrich's lower fat content and quick cooking time make it ideal for a vegetable stir-fry supper. Cook quickly and DO NOT overcook.

1	1b ostrich filets, cut into 1½" pieces
2	Tbsp coconut oil
2	med garlic cloves, sliced
1	1" piece ginger, sliced
1	small leek, washed and cut into rings
4	cups shredded Chinese cabbage
8	oz button mushrooms, halved
1	med red pepper, cut into strips
1	10 oz pkg fresh snow peas, cut in half, diagonally
1	Tbsp tamari soy sauce

Nutrition Facts

	calories	*total fat*	*carbs*	*protein*
Mixed Type:	300	12g	11g	38g
Carb Type:	221	7g	11g	29g
Protein Type:	338	19g	12g	32g

Cooking Tips

PT: Substitute grass-fed beef filet or strip steak for ostrich. Increase mushrooms to 12 oz.

CT: Reduce ostrich to 12 oz. Reduce coconut oil to 1 Tbsp.

Notes and Suggestions

Lowfat ostrich and vegetables are a great combination for a CT. You could also serve a salad with this, or a soup such as Fast French Onion.

1 heat wok or deep heavy porcelain-clad skillet over medium high heat. Add coconut oil, garlic, ginger, and leek slices. Sauté until leeks starts to wilt.

2 add ostrich meat and sauté for 1–2 minutes. Remove meat from pan and hold, covered. Remove ginger slices.

3 add Chinese cabbage and mushroom halves to pan and stir-fry until cabbage starts to wilt. Add red pepper strips and snow peas. Stir-fry for 1–2 minutes more. Add already cooked ostrich.

4 remove from heat. Add soy sauce and stir to combine. Serve immediately.

Serves 4. Preparation time: 15 minutes.

Red Peppery Buffalo Steaks

Buffalo steaks with a crusty kick of crushed peppercorns, lemon and salt, served over braised Chinese cabbage with an easy roasted pepper sauce.

1	lb bison ribeye steaks
2–3	Tbsp dried green and black peppercorns
1	tsp coarse sea salt
1	tsp grated lemon zest
4	cups Chinese cabbage, ¼" diagonal cuts
1	med garlic clove, smashed
8	oz jar roasted red peppers
1	tsp tamari soy sauce or Spike vegetable seasoning

1 crush peppercorns with back of spoon or in grinder. Mix with sea salt and lemon zest. Press mixture all over steaks. Let marinate with this coating for at least a few minutes. More flavor, if allowed to penetrate for 30 minutes.

2 sear steaks by broiling in oven broiler, over the grill, or in heavy cast iron skillet on medium high heat, 3 minutes on a side. If frying, remove steaks from pan. Add shredded Chinese cabbage and garlic to pan drippings and stir-fry until wilted.

3 meanwhlile, blend roasted red peppers in blender with 1 tsp tamari soy sauce or Spike vegetable seasoning.

4 to assemble, pile serving platter with braised cabbage, top with steaks and pour red pepper sauce over top. Serve immediately.

Serves 4. Preparation time: 15 minutes.

Nutrition Facts

	calories	total fat	carbs	protein
Mixed Type:	158	3g	6g	27g
Carb Type:	134	3g	6g	22g
Protein Type:	232	4g	13g	37g

Cooking Tips

PT: You could substitute cauliflower for cabbage and serve 3 with this recipe.

CT: Bison or buffalo is not a recommended meat for your type. But you could use this recipe, substituting ostrich steaks, reducing quantity to 12 oz.

Notes and Suggestions

This is a timesaving version of the classic pepper steak recipe. These steaks go well with Mashed Fotatoes or Roasted Asparagus.

Nutrition Facts

	calories	total fat	carbs	protein
Mixed Type:	384	8g	48g	30g
Carb Type:	322	4g	48g	21g
Protein Type:	380	9g	15g	57g

Cooking Tips

PT: Increase meat to 2 lb. Increase celery to 6 stalks. Substitute 2 Tbsp dried cherries or currants for cranberries. Serve to 4.

CT: Reduce coconut oil to 1 1/2 tsp. Use 1 lb venison. Use 3 kohlrabi and add 3 cups chopped cabbage with vegetables before covering and simmering.

Notes and Suggestions

Serve this hearty stew as a special treat over Mashed Fotatoes or Braised Fennel.

Venison Stew

Lower fat wild or organic meats like venison are especially good in stews where they can be cooked in liquid.

1 1/2	lb wild or organic stewing venison
	sea salt and pepper
1	Tbsp coconut oil or butter
1	med red onion, sliced
3	stalks celery, cut diagonally
2	tsp thyme leaves
1	tsp ground cinnamon
1	tsp grated orange peel (no white)
1/2	cup fresh cranberries
3	med kohlrabi, peeled and chopped
3	cups natural beef stock

1 season venison with salt and pepper.

2 in large stockpot or porcelain-clad Dutch oven over medium heat, sauté onion and celery in coconut oil until onion starts to become translucent. Remove vegetables and hold.

3 add venison meat and sear or cook until browned and sealed. Add thyme leaves, cinnamon, orange peel. Stir to distribute. Add cranberries, kohlrabi, sautéed vegetables and stock.

4 heat until mixture starts to bubble. Cover and simmer at medium low for 45–50 minutes or until venison is tender. Serve.

Serves 6. Preparation time: 15 minutes.

Basic Roast Chicken

A simple, basic poultry recipe is the classic Sunday Roast Chicken.

1	6–8 lb free range roasting chicken
1	Tbsp raw or organic butter, softened
1	med garlic clove, minced
3/4	tsp sea salt
4–5	grinds freshly ground black pepper
2	tsp thyme leaves

1 preheat oven to 350°F. Wash chicken, removing fat from inside cavity.

2 in small bowl, combine butter, minced garlic, salt, pepper and thyme leaves. Rub this paste over outside of chicken. Place bird breast-side-down in roasting pan.

3 roast, uncovered, basting frequently, for approximately $1\frac{1}{2}$ hours, (about 20 minutes per pound). Place chicken breast-side-up during last half an hour to brown.

4 remove from oven when leg pulls easily and juices no longer run red. Remove from pan and let rest, covered, for 5–10 minutes. Deglaze or scrape pan juices and make gravy, if desired, from $1\frac{1}{2}$ Tbsp arrowroot, dissolved in two cups water.

5 cut chicken into servings or slice and serve with gravy on the side. Remove skin before eating. Remove leftover chicken from bone and refrigerate or freeze for expediting meals during the week.

Serves 11. Preparation time: 10 minutes.

Nutrition Facts

	calories	total fat	carbs	protein
Mixed Type:	215	8g	0g	33g
Carb Type:	196	5g	0g	35g
Protein Type:	232	11g	0g	31g

Cooking Tips

MX: Choose half dark & half white meat portions.

PT: Choose dark meat portions.

CT: Choose white meat portions.

Notes and Suggestions

Roasting a chicken or turkey is a basic skill everyone needs to know. A standby you can count on for a no-fail Sunday dinner, roasting a bird at the beginning of the week assures a good supply of ready-to-eat protein for lunches and dinners during the week. Add cooked meat as the protein complement for soups, salads, casseroles, fillings, egg dishes, Roll-Ups and "sandwiches."

Nutrition Facts

	calories	total fat	carbs	protein
Mixed Type:	260	13g	1g	33g
Carb Type:	239	10g	1g	35g
Protein Type:	275	16g	1g	31g

Cooking Tips

PT: Choose 5 oz. dark meat portions. Use 2 cups BBQ sauce.

CT: Use 1 cup BBQ sauce. Serve 3 oz white meat portions.

Notes and Suggestions

This is not your typical sweet and sticky BBQ chicken, but this classic recipe, developed by Cornell Cooperative Extension, has withstood the test of time. This is excellent served with Grilled Ratatouille Salad, which you can make right along with the chicken on the grill. Despite continual basting, not all of the sauce will be used. Unused BBQ sauce (that was not used to marinate raw chicken) can be kept in the refrigerator in covered glass jar for up to 8 weeks.

Classic Cornell BBQ Chicken

Without a doubt, the BEST non-tomato barbecue sauce going. Savory, piquant and pungent, but not spicy or sweet. No wonder it's been popular for almost 50 years!

4	broiler-fryer halves
1½	cups Cornell BBQ Sauce (page 242)

1 marinate broiler-fryer halves in BBQ sauce, turning occasionally, for up to 8 hours.

2 heat up grill or preheat broiler. Grilling is definitely the best. Cook chicken, liberally and frequently basting with BBQ sauce. Turn halves routinely, on outdoor grill for approximately 1½ hours until tender and dark brown.

3 cut each half into 2–3 portions, depending upon eating plan. Four broiler-fryer halves will generally feed 8–10 of all except the biggest eaters. Serve immediately.

4 can be prepared in the broiler/oven, reducing cooking time, but there's no comparison with the grilled product. Excellent leftover, cold, if there is any.

Serves 8–10. Preparation time: 10 minutes.

Crockpot Turkey Stew

A warm, welcoming fall or winter one-dish-meal waiting for you in the crockpot when you get home.

2	lb free-range turkey parts
1	med leek, sliced
2	stalks celery, cut into pieces
2	tsp thyme leaves
1	tsp oregano leaves
1	tsp Spike or Mrs Dash vegetable seasoning
1	cup winter squash, peeled and cubed
1	med carrot, chopped
1	cinnamon stick
1	16 oz can tomatoes
2	cups water or free-range chicken stock
1	cup lentil or mung bean sprouts

1 place turkey pieces, skin-side-down, into crockpot set on high, and sauté to release fat. Turn turkey pieces and add leeks and celery. Sprinkle on thyme, oregano and vegetable seasoning, and sauté until leeks start to become translucent.

2 add squash cubes, carrots, cinnamon stick, tomatoes, water or stock, and simmer covered, for 2–3 hours on medium or up to 6–8 hours on lowest setting.

3 a few minutes before serving, add lentil or bean sprouts and remove cinnamon stick. Serve immediately.

Serves 4. Preparation time: 15 minutes.

Nutrition Facts

	calories	total fat	carbs	protein
Mixed Type:	252	9g	25g	21g
Carb Type:	254	4g	44g	15g
Protein Type:	284	10g	24g	25g

Cooking Tips

PT: Increase celery to 4 stalks. Substitute kohlrabi for squash. Use dark meat turkey such as legs and thighs.

CT: Use 1 lb turkey breast meat. Use 1–28 oz can tomatoes. Reduce cooking time to 1 hour.

Notes and Suggestions

This is close to a one-dish-meal, but you could easily pair it with a quick vegetable like Sautéed Cabbage with Dill or Braised Brazilian Greens to have dinner on the table in a few minutes.

Crunchy Chicken Salad / Casserole

This convertible chicken salad-to-casserole is a tasty way to use up leftover cooked chicken or turkey.

3	cups leftover cooked free-range chicken
2	cups coarsely diced celery
2	Tbsp chopped green onions
1	cup jicama, peeled and cut into matchsticks
2	tsp lemon juice
²/₃	cup basic mayonnaise (page 238)
¼	cup walnuts, coarsely chopped
½	tsp sea salt
½	tsp freshly ground black pepper
3	dashes Angoustura bitters (optional)
	lettuce or spinach leaves (optional)

1 in large bowl or lightly greased casserole, mix all ingredients together until combined.

2 to serve as salad, refrigerate or serve immediately on lettuce or spinach leaves.

3 to serve as casserole, preheat oven to 350°F. Transfer chicken salad to lightly greased casserole dish. Top with 1 Tbsp Sunny Seed Gomasio (page 215) or Parmesan cheese. Bake for 15–18 minutes until warmed through.

Serves 5. Preparation time: 10 minutes.

Nutrition Facts

	calories	total fat	carbs	protein
Mixed Type:	197	10g	5g	22g
Carb Type:	170	7g	9g	22g
Protein Type:	260	14g	6g	27g

Cooking Tips

PT: Use 4 cups dark meat chicken. Increase celery to 3 cups and walnuts to ¹/₃ cup.

CT: Use 2 cups white meat chicken. Use ¹/₃ cup mayonnaise and ¹/₃ cup plain lowfat yogurt. Reduce walnuts to 2 Tbsp, combined with 2 Tbsp chopped parsley and sprinkled on top.

Notes and Suggestions

This is a hearty standalone lunch or summer supper meal, with the appropriate type of light or dark meat poultry for your type. Serve on lettuce leaves or small mound of spinach for PT. CT's can also serve this with a mixed vegetable side salad lightly tossed with Basic Herb Vinaigrette (page 237).

Grilled Caribbean Rub

Dry rubs are a simple, yet very flavorful way to season meats with fewer calories and carbs.

2	free-range broiler-fryer halves
1	Tbsp coconut oil or raw organic butter
6	Tbsp Caribbean Jerk Rub

Caribbean Jerk Rub — Mix together:

6	Tbsp minced garlic or garlic powder
6	Tbsp minced onion,
6	Tbsp dried minced onion or onion powder,
2	Tbsp allspice
1	Tbsp dried ground chipotle or red pepper,
2	Tbsp Hungarian paprika,
1	packet SteviaPlus alternative sweetener Or
1	Tbsp dried organic cane juice
2	Tbsp thyme leaves,
2	Tbsp ground cinnamon, 2 tsp ground nutmeg
1½	tsp ground habeñera,
	ground zest or peel of 2 lemons (no white)

Store in covered container in refrigerator, for up to a month.

1 heat up grill or preheat broiler.

2 rub broiler-fryer halves lightly with oil and then all over with Jerk Rub.

3 broil or grill, turning routinely, until chicken is tender, approximately 1 to 1½ hours.

Serves 5. Preparation time: 10 minutes.

Nutrition Facts

	calories	total fat	carbs	protein
Mixed Type:	215	8g	0g	33g
Carb Type:	196	5g	0g	35g
Protein Type:	232	11g	0g	31g

Cooking Tips

PT: Select dark meat portions.

CT: Select white meat portions. Serve 6. CT's may want to remove skin just before cooking is done, as it is high in fat. Sprinkle additional Jerk Rub over meat to increase flavor, if desired.

Notes and Suggestions

A quick, no-fuss chicken preparation for fast supper or backyard grilling. Combine with a Grilled Ratatouille Salad or a tossed garden vegetable salad with crunchy toppings for a whole meal.

Grilled Chicken Caesar

A classic chicken meal salad, made even more special with grilled chicken.

2	whole free-range chicken breasts, split
1/2	tsp Spike vegetable seasoning or Mrs. Dash
1/2	tsp freshly ground black pepper
1	large head Romaine lettuce, torn
1	Tbsp capers
1/4	cup Caesar salad dressing
1/4	cup grated Parmesan or Romano cheese

Nutrition Facts

	calories	total fat	carbs	protein
Mixed Type:	265	11g	9g	32g
Carb Type:	200	6g	5g	30g
Protein Type:	300	20g	8g	22g

Cooking Tips

PT: Use 4 lbs chicken thighs. Substitute 4 cups spinach for 4 cups of the lettuce. Add 2 cups chopped celery.

CT: Use 2 Tbsp capers, 2 Tbsp salad dressing and 2 Tbsp Parmesan cheese.

Notes and Suggestions

An excellent summer meal salad to make with leftover grilled or broiled chicken. PT's could also accompany it with Parmesan Crisps.

1 preheat broiler. Cut split breast halves crosswise in 1" slices. Season with Spike and pepper. Broil chicken pieces on slatted broiler tray 3-6 minutes, or until golden brown. Remove from oven and cool.

2 meanwhile, wash and drain romaine. Tear into large pieces into salad bowl.

3 add remaining ingredients, except for 2 Tbsp Parmesan cheese, and toss until coated. Top with broiled chicken pieces and remaining Parmesan cheese.

Serves 4. Preparation time: 10 minutes.

Ground Turkey and Gravy

A quick, satisfying dish when there's little time left to get a meal on the table.

1	small onion, chopped
1	lb free-range ground turkey
8	oz button mushrooms, quartered
2	tsp thyme leaves
2	Tbsp Beans 'R' Us bean flour, arrowroot or soy flour (page 252)
2	cups clean, filtered water
1	Tbsp tamari soy sauce

1 heat medium skillet over medium high. Add onions and dry sauté for a few minutes.

2 add ground turkey, mushrooms, and thyme leaves, and sauté until pink of meat is gone, about 5–6 minutes.

3 add flour and stir to coat, heating for 20–30 seconds. Add water, stir and cook, stirring frequently, until mixture is thickened. Remove from heat and stir in soy sauce.

4 serve immediately as is, over Mashed Fotatoes, Zuchetti Pasta, or Spaghetti Squash.

Serves 4. Preparation time: 10 minutes.

Nutrition Facts

	calories	total fat	carbs	protein
Mixed Type:	232	13g	5g	23g
Carb Type:	200	10g	12g	17g
Protein Type:	281	16g	6g	29g

Cooking Tips

PT: Increase turkey to $1^1/4$ lb. Increase mushrooms to 12 oz.

CT: Reduce oil to 2 tsp. Reduce turkey to 12 oz. Use 1 med sliced onion. Add $^1/2$ chopped green pepper and 6 oz water chestnut slices after meat is cooked.

Notes and Suggestions

This is a very good dish to serve over Mashed Fotatoes or Zucchetti Pasta, accompanied by a green salad for a whole meal.

Hot Wings, Thighs & Things

Everybody's favorite snack while watching the game, now you don't have to miss out.

2	lb free-range chicken parts, wings, thighs and breasts
1¹/₂	cups commercial chicken wing sauce
¹/₂	tsp Tabasco sauce
¹/₂	tsp freshly ground black pepper
¹/₄	cup sesame seeds
6	large celery stalks, cut into sticks
¹/₂	cup blue cheese dressing

Nutrition Facts

	calories	total fat	carbs	protein
Mixed Type:	274	24g	8g	10g
Carb Type:	170	11g	5g	8g
Protein Type:	324	27g	8g	11g

Cooking Tips

PT: Use dark meat such as wings and thighs. Increase celery sticks to 12 and blue cheese dressing to ²/₃ cup.

CT: Serve this recipe using white meat chicken. Reduce blue cheese dressing to ¹/₃ cup and omit sesame seeds.

Notes and Suggestions

Most commercial chicken wing sauce is low in carbs. You can serve this with Rainbow Cabbage Salad or Vegetable Crispers, or a big plate of raw vegetable dippers with lots of celery.

1 preheat oven to 375°F. Wash chicken and drain. Cut up chicken into large nugget-type pieces. Place chicken in 9" x 13" baking pan.

2 drench chicken with hot wings sauce, mixed with Tabasco and pepper. Sprinkle all over with sesame seeds.

3 bake for 20–25 minutes, until meat is cooked through or reads 165°F. Remove from oven and transfer to serving platter.

4 surround Hot Wings & Things with celery sticks and a small dipping bowl of blue cheese dressing.

Serves 4. Preparation time: 10 minutes.

Quick Turkey Cutlets

Another tasty turkey dish that could help get dinner on the table in a hurry any weeknight.

1¼	lb boned free-range turkey thighs
1¼	tsp sea or celtic sea salt
4–5	grinds freshly ground black pepper
¼	cup lemon juice
4	tsp raw or organic butter or coconut oil
4	tsp fresh minced or 2 tsp crushed dried rosemary
2	Tbsp green olives, sliced in half

1 place boned turkey thighs between pieces of waxed paper or plastic wrap and pound with large flat knife or meat mallet evenly to ⅛" thick. Sprinkle with salt and pepper.

2 heat 12" sauté pan or large skillet over medium high heat until hot. Melt butter and sear turkey cutlets quickly, until browned. Turn cutlets. Cook for 1 minute.

3 sprinkle with rosemary and add lemon juice and olives. Cook for 2–3 minutes more. Then remove cutlets to serving platter and keep warm.

4 continue heating sauce while deglazing or scraping up any browned bits from bottom of pan until sauce is reduced to about 2 Tbsp. Pour over turkey cutlets on platter and serve immediately.

Serves 4. Preparation time: 10 minutes.

Nutrition Facts

	calories	total fat	carbs	protein
Mixed Type:	275	13g	4g	36g
Carb Type:	210	6g	4g	30g
Protein Type:	387	15g	5g	50g

Cooking Tips

PT: This is an ideal dish for you as is. Use 3 Tbsp olives, if desired.

CT: Light meat turkey breast is more appropriate for your type. Start with 1 lb, 2 half breast portions, cut in half and flattened as directed. Reduce butter to 2 tsp. Omit olives and substitute 2 tsp capers.

Notes and Suggestions

This quick turkey entrée could be a fast supper on a night when there's no time to fuss. Serve it with steamed green beans, asparagus, or leftover broccoli slaw if you are a PT. CT can serve with a mixed green salad with Basic Herb Vinaigrette or Braised Cabbage with Dill.

Roast Turkey with Vegetable Chestnut Stuffing

A garlic, vegetable, and herb stuffing assures moistness and gives this turkey a rich, savory flavor.

1	13–14 lb free-range turkey
1	Tbsp raw butter or coconut oil
5	med garlic cloves, minced
2	large onions, chopped
8	large stalks celery, chopped
2	med carrots, coarsely shredded
2	med kohlrabi, peeled and chopped
2	med green apple, finely chopped
3	cups chopped Italian flat-leaf parsley, packed
2	cups coarsely chopped chestnuts or sliced water chestnuts
1	Tbsp black currants
2	Tbsp poultry seasoning or
1	Tbsp thyme leaves, 2 tsp sage leaves, $3/4$ tsp crushed rosemary
1	tsp sea or celtic sea salt
$1/2$	tsp freshly ground black pepper

Nutrition Facts

	calories	total fat	carbs	protein
Mixed Type:	289	7g	37g	19g
Carb Type:	215	3g	33g	15g
Protein Type:	310	9g	37g	19g

Cooking Tips

PT: Choose dark meat. If you prefer, you can omit the fruits and add $1^1/2$ lb sliced mushrooms at the end while cooking the vegetables.

CT: Choose breast meat. Choose water chestnuts instead of chestnuts for stuffing. Serve smaller portions to 24.

Notes and Suggestions

Yes, it's also possible for you to enjoy the traditional Thanksgiving and/or Christmas turkey dinner with the trimmings—even the stuffing—and still maintain your eating plan. Just watch your portions. Those who have diabetes or obesity may wish to forgo the stuffing due to high carb count.

1 remove giblets and neck. Rinse turkey inside and out. Rub with 1 tsp butter or coconut oil. Sprinkle with salt and pepper. Preheat oven to 350°F.

2 in large kettle or pot, melt remaining butter or coconut oil. Add minced garlic and onions and sauté until vegetables are translucent. Add celery, carrots, kohlrabi, and apple and sauté until vegetables start to soften. Remove from heat.

3 add chopped parsley and chestnuts or water chestnuts, currants, poultry seasoning, salt and pepper. Mix together well.

4 stuff turkey, tie back legs. Place breast-side-down in shallow roasting pan. Cover with aluminum foil. Roast for 1 hour. Reduce temperature to 200°F. Roast for 2 hours.

5 turn bird breast-side-up and and roast for an additional 2 hours and 45 minutes or until internal temperature of thighs reaches 160–170°F. Remove bird from oven. Increase oven temperature to 400°F, remove foil and return bird to oven for an additional 10 minutes until thigh temperature reaches 170°F. and breast skin is brown.

6 remove turkey from oven and allow to rest on cutting board for 20 minutes before carving. Scoop out stuffing and put into serving bowl, covered, until it's time to eat. Slice turkey and serve.

Serves 20. Preparation time: 25 minutes.

Roasted Tomatillo Turkey Salad

Leftover turkey goes south of the border in a quick, healthy meal salad with smoky crunch.

3	cups cooked, boned, free-range turkey, cut up
1	cup cubed jicama
½	cup finely chopped celery
½	cup finely chopped broccoli stems
2	med scallions or green onions, sliced
¼	cup pimento-stuffed green olives, chopped
½	cup chopped cilantro or Italian flat-leaf parsley
3	Tbsp lemon juice
½	cup Green Olive Tomatillo Salsa (page 243)
4–5	grinds fresh black pepper

1 combine cooked turkey, jicama, celery, broccoli stems, scallions, green olives, cilantro or flat-leaf parsley in large mixing bowl.

2 stir lemon juice into green olive salsa. Pour over salad. Toss to combine. Serve on butter lettuce leaves.

Serves 4. Preparation time: 5 minutes.

Nutrition Facts

	calories	total fat	carbs	protein
Mixed Type:	299	14g	11g	31g
Carb Type:	233	9g	8g	22g
Protein Type:	388	24g	12g	40g

Cooking Tips

PT: Increase turkey to 4 cups dark meat. Increase celery to 1½ cups. Increase olives to ⅓ cup.

CT: Substitute white meat turkey and reduce to 2 cups. Omit olives.

Notes and Suggestions

This is a unique salad that could be made easily from leftover turkey. It can also be made easily into a soup with the simple addition of hot chicken broth. Find the recipe on page 136 in Soups.

Slowdown Crockpot Chicken Curry

This could cook while you're away during the day, then be almost ready to serve when you return. Simple and Fast... You're not standing there watching the crockpot, are you?

2	lb free-range chicken parts
1	small onion cut into rings or 1/2" pieces
3	large celery stalks, cut into 2" diagonal cuts
3	garlic cloves, minced
1	Tbsp curry powder
1/4	tsp cayenne pepper
	salt and pepper
2	Tbsp Beans 'R' Us bean flour, soy flour or arrowroot (page 252)
1/2	cup half and half cream or buttermilk
	broth from cooking chicken

1 in crockpot, place chicken pieces, onion, celery, garlic, curry powder, cayenne, salt and pepper. Cook on low for 5–6 hours.

2 remove chicken from crockpot to colander set in a large bowl. Let drain and cool slightly. Remove chicken from bones. Reserve stock.

3 combine remaining liquid from crockpot with 2 Tbsp bean flour in a medium saucepan. Bring to a boil and cook until mixture thickens slightly.

4 reduce heat, add half and half or buttermilk, cooked chicken meat, and additional curry to taste.

5 serve with any combination of traditional curry accompaniments such as: cooked, crumbled turkey bacon, chopped scallion or green onion tops, fresh or dried, unsweetened coconut, mung bean sprouts, chopped hard-cooked egg, chopped walnuts, and/or currants. Choose 2, about 1 Tbsp each.

Serves 4. Preparation time: 15 minutes.

Nutrition Facts

	calories	total fat	carbs	protein
Mixed Type:	241	6g	8g	37g
Carb Type:	222	3g	9g	37g
Protein Type:	361	13g	7g	49g

Cooking Tips

PT: Can increase celery to 5 large stalks. Use dark meat portions. Choose half and half cream over buttermilk

CT: Use white meat and lowfat buttermilk. Cook only 1 hour maximum.

Notes and Suggestions

This dish could be the centerpiece for an Asian or Indian-inspired meal.

Steaming Chicken and Vegetables

Steaming the chicken with vegetables is a simple, healthy method that reduces excess fat, cooking time and kitchen mess.

1	med head savoy cabbage, shredded
3/4	cup baby carrots, split in half
1	1" piece fresh ginger root, sliced and cut into matchsticks
1	med garlic clove, minced
6	scallions or green onions, cut into thirds
1/2	cup Italian or flat-leaf parsley, lightly chopped
1	tsp sea salt or Spike vegetable seasoning
3–4	grinds fresh black pepper
2	large chicken breasts, halved
2	tsp coconut oil or butter
1/2	cup free-range chicken stock

1 the preferable utensil for steaming this dish is a bundt pan (the cake pan with a hole in the middle). However, it could be done in a bamboo steamer or a regular metal colander with legs in a covered stockpot.

2 bring 2–3 inches of water to boil in large Dutch oven or stockpot. Place shredded cabbage in bottom of bundt pan or steamer basket. Lower heat under water to simmer.

3 meanwhile, combine sliced carrots, ginger, garlic, scallions, parsley, and chicken in a large bowl. Add oil, sprinkle with salt or Spike and pepper. Toss to mix. Pile mixture evenly on top of shredded cabbage.

4 place steamer/pan into stockpot of simmering water. Pour chicken stock over, cover and steam lightly for about 18–20 minutes.

Serves 4. Preparation time: 15 minutes.

Nutrition Facts

	calories	total fat	carbs	protein
Mixed Type:	225	4g	16g	31g
Carb Type:	218	4g	16g	29g
Protein Type:	242	5g	14g	36g

Cooking Tips

PT: Use 2 1/2 lb dark meat chicken, thigh, wings and/or legs, instead of breast meat. Could substitute 2 cups asparagus or green bean cuts for 2 cups of the cabbage.

CT: Use chicken breasts. Can increase parsley to 1 cup. Add 1 cup red or yellow pepper strips, if desired.

Notes and Suggestions

Another standalone meal in itself, this is an ideal dish for any type, but especially CT. Here's a good example of a dish that is light and healthy with a good balance of protein and vegetables. Yet, PT and even MX may find that this doesn't have enough fat to keep from getting hungry soon after eating. If so, you could serve with one of the Extra's in Condiments, like Black Olive Tapenade, Chunky Mockamole or Miso Walnut Paste.

Stir-Fry Turkey

This is the basic recipe for the fast Oriental wonder, Stir-Fry. In traditional wok or heavy skillet, over gas, electric or open fire, this is the mother of all fast and healthy meals in a minute.

1	Tbsp coconut oil, raw or organic butter
3	slices ginger root
1	large garlic clove, sliced
1	med red onion, chopped
2	cups celery, diagonally cut
1	med carrot, cut in half slices
1	broccoli stem, peeled and sliced
2	med kohlrabi, peeled and diced
1	cup broccoli flowerettes
3	cups chopped kale or spinach
8	oz mushrooms, sliced or quartered
2	cups cooked leftover turkey or chicken
2	tsp dried thyme or marjoram leaves
1/4	tsp curry powder
1	Tbsp tamari soy sauce

Nutrition Facts

	calories	total fat	carbs	protein
Mixed Type:	250	8g	20g	28g
Carb Type:	237	7g	20g	27g
Protein Type:	366	14g	20g	42g

Cooking Tips

PT: Choose or use as many of the recommended vegetables for your type as possible—particularly green beans, cauliflower, celery, mushrooms, and spinach. Choose preferred meats such as dark meat chicken or turkey, beef, bison, lamb, venison, or even salmon. Increase dark meat to 3½ cups and increase mushrooms to 12 oz.

CT: Opt for the recommended vegetables and light meats on your list.

Notes and Suggestions

This basic stir-fry technique can be used with almost kind of vegetables and meats. So this is an ideal, versatile recipe that allows you the choice of vegetables and cuts of meat that work best for your metabolic type. The whole secret with this speedy meal-in-one preparation is to have everything cut up in equal size pieces, close at hand and ready before you fire up the heat. Then with heat on HIGH and constant stirring, the vegetables are added in sequence, starting with the densest first. Once practiced, it's literally possible to have a complete one dish dinner on the table in less than 10 minutes!

1 make sure all vegetables are cut up and ingredients are close at hand. Heat spun steel wok or heavy porcelain-clad casserole over high heat. When hot, add coconut oil, ginger root and sliced garlic, stirring constantly for about 30–45 seconds.

2 add onion, celery, carrot, broccoli stems, kohlrabi, and stir-fry, stirring constantly, for 3–4 minutes, or until vegetable colors brighten.

3 add broccoli flowerettes, kale, and mushrooms, and continue to stir-fry for 1 minute.

4 add cooked turkey, dried herbs and curry powder. Cover, reduce heat to medium low, and let steam finish cooking for about 2 minutes. Shut off heat. Remove cover, stir in tamari and serve immediately.

5 if using uncooked meat or poultry, add uniformly cut up pieces after the dense vegetables are cooking for a couple of minutes. If adding already-cooked meat, add at the end, as described.

Serves 4. Preparation time: 15 minutes.

Tarragon Turkey Burgers

These are delicious! And not much more trouble than making regular burgers.

1	lb free-range ground turkey
1/2	cup coarsely shredded zucchini
1/4	cup chopped red onion
1	Tbsp fresh or dried tarragon leaves
2	tsp Dijon mustard
1/2	tsp Spike vegetable seasoning or sea salt
3	grinds fresh black pepper
2	large eggs

1 preheat broiler. In mixing bowl, combine ground turkey with zucchini, onion, tarragon, mustard, Spike, pepper, and eggs. Mix thoroughly.

2 shape into patties. Place on broiler pan. Broil 5 minutes on a side until browned. Serve immediately.

Serves 4. Preparation time: 5 minutes.

Nutrition Facts

	calories	total fat	carbs	protein
Mixed Type:	216	12g	2g	23g
Carb Type:	221	12g	3g	24g
Protein Type:	259	14g	2g	28g

Cooking Tips

PT: Increase ground turkey to $1^1/4$ lb and Dijon mustard to 1 Tbsp. Substitute finely chopped celery for zucchini.

CT: Increase zucchini to $^3/4$ cup and red onion to $^1/2$ cup. Add another teaspoon of Dijon mustard.

Notes and Suggestions

These burgers are so popular, even teenagers love them. Pair with a green bean casserole or steamed Broccoli-in-a-Hurry Curry for a great meal.

Cauliflower Tempeh Curry

This hearty, luxurious combination of flavors and textures will satisfy even non-vegetarians.

1	Tbsp coconut oil
1/2	cup chopped onions
2	med garlic cloves
2	med kohlrabi, peeled, sliced and quartered
2	heaping cups cauliflowerettes
1	cup diced zucchini
2	Tbsp curry powder
1/2	tsp ground cinnamon
2	mild green chilies, seeded and chopped
1	16 oz can lite coconut milk
1	10 oz pkg tempeh, cut into 1/2" pieces
1/2	cup raw cashews
	tamari soy sauce

Nutrition Facts

	calories	total fat	carbs	protein
Mixed Type:	425	30g	28g	21g
Carb Type:	393	29g	23g	19g
Protein Type:	463	37g	26g	17g

Cooking Tips

PT: PT's really need meat in their meals, so you could add some cooked chicken to this in place of part of the tempeh.

CT: Use 1/4 cup shaved coconut in place of cashews. Reduce coconut milk to 1 cup.

Notes and Suggestions

This a one-dish-meal could be satisfying in itself for a CT, and with additional meat protein for a PT. If you are PT and want or are trying to follow a vegetarian meal plan, you will have to be honest with yourself in monitoring how you feel and realize that PT's have a high requirement for protein that generally cannot be met through vegetable sources alone. Especially since most vegetarian diets these days usually rely upon a larger proportion of soyfood, not as healthy as has been touted (see page 18 for details). Once again, the key is to honestly observe and monitor how your body feels after eating.

1 heat a large skillet over medium high. Add 1 Tbsp coconut oil, onions, garlic and sauté until onions are translucent. Add kohlrabi cuts, cauliflowerettes, diced zucchini, and continue cooking for a few more minutes.

2 add curry, cinnamon, chilies, and coconut milk, stirring to combine. Cover and simmer 10 minutes, until you have finished browning tempeh, next step.

3 in a smaller skillet, heat 1 Tbsp coconut oil, add tempeh pieces and sauté, stirring frequently, over medium heat, until tempeh pieces are golden. Remove from heat and splash with tamari soy sauce.

4 either add the tempeh to the curried vegetables and stir to combine, or pile tempeh pieces on top of vegetables in serving bowl. Sprinkle with cashews. Serve immediately.

Serves 4. Preparation time: 20 minutes.

Eggplant Cheeseburgers

These "burgers," though not as dense, look and taste good, like their original counterparts.

1	med eggplant, sliced into $1/2$" – $3/4$" slices
2	tsp sea salt
2	med whole egg (for dipping)
$1^{1}/_{2}$	Tbsp tahini, sesame seed butter, thinned with 1 Tbsp water
$1/4$	cup Sunny Seed Gomasio (page 219)
1	tsp coconut oil
1	med thinly sliced tomato
1	small red onion, sliced into thin rings
$1/2$	cup raw, grass-fed shredded mozzarella, cheddar, Swiss or provolone cheese
	lettuce or green cabbage leaves

1 sprinkle eggplant slices with salt. Let stand until salt draws out bitter liquid. Rinse off salt and pat dry.

2 beat eggs or add water to sesame seed butter to thin. Dip eggplant into egg or sesame tahini, then roll in seed mixture, coating both sides.

3 heat a large skillet over medium heat. Melt coconut oil and tilt pan to distribute evenly. Sauté eggplant slices 4–5 minute, or until they start to brown.

4 carefully turn slices with spatula. Top with tomato and red onion slice. Sprinkle with cheese. Continue cooking until second side is golden and cheese melts.

5 serve on large platter or "sandwich" cheeseburgers between lettuce or cabbage leaves to replace the bun.

Serves 4. Preparation time: 20 minutes.

Nutrition Facts

	calories	total fat	carbs	protein
Mixed Type:	169	10g	13g	10g
Carb Type:	127	7g	13g	7g

Cooking Tips

PT: Protein Types need to eat some meat protein at almost all meals, and eggplant is not one of your top recommended veggies, so this is not the best recipe for you.

CT: Depending upon how well you handle dairy products, you could substitute grated Parmesan or use a little lowfat ricotta for your cheese. Otherwise, go for "plain" burgers.

Notes and Suggestions

You could pair this with KISS Salad in a Flash, or a light soup for a whole meal.

Mushroom Burgers

These hearty burgers are surprisingly tasty AND satisfying, without meat.

¹/₂	cup finely chopped red onion
2	cups Portabella mushrooms, cut into chunks
¹/₂	cup finely chopped pecans, walnuts or macadamia nuts
¹/₂	cup chopped parsley
¹/₂	cup coarsely shredded zucchini, patted dry
1	tsp marjoram leaves
2	tsp thyme leaves
2	tsp tamari soy sauce
¹/₃	cup shredded grassfed Swiss or jack cheese
3	med eggs, beaten
3	Tbsp Sunny Seed Gomasio (page 215)
2	Tbsp coconut oil for frying

1 combine onions, mushroom chunks, chopped nuts, chopped parsley, zucchini, marjoram and thyme leaves, soy sauce, shredded cheese, and eggs.

2 shape by hand into patties. Coat both sides with ground seed Gomasio in a small bowl.

3 heat a medium skillet over medium. Melt coconut oil. Pan fry "burgers" 3–4 minutes per side, until golden brown. Serve immediately.

Serves 4. Preparation time: 15 minutes.

Nutrition Facts

	calories	total fat	carbs	protein
Mixed Type:	344	25g	19g	17g
Carb Type:	221	11g	19g	17g

Cooking Tips

PT: PT's need to get meat protein in their meals. Not an ideal recipe for you.

CT: Substitute grated soy tempeh for nuts. Reduce cheese to ¹/4 cup shredded Parmesan. Reduce oil to 2 tsp for frying.

Notes and Suggestions

Serve these patties with a tossed salad and some Vegetable Crispers for a healthy, "fast food-like" meal.

No-Pasta Primavera

This updated version of the classic, seasonal, Italian vegetable pasta can be ladled over spaghetti squash or zucchini "pasta" for a satisfying summer meal.

1	**large spaghetti squash, cooked**
1	**Recipe No-Pasta Primavera Vegetables (page 171)**
¼	**cup Parmesan cheese**
¼	**cup Savory Sunny Seed Mix, optional (page 215)**

1 fill large 6-quart porcelain-clad Dutch oven or large saucepan ⅔'s full with water and bring to a boil.

2 holding squash carefully, cut spaghetti squash in half with cleaver or heavy knife. Lay cut side down and cut in half again, yielding four pieces. Add to pot and simmer covered, for about 20 minutes, until squash separates into "strings" or strands with fork. Remove from heat and drain. Scoop out squash quarter and place squash in covered serving dish. Keep warm.

3 while squash is cooking, prepare No-Pasta Primavera Vegetables found in Vegetables chapter.

4 serve immediately as is, or topped with Parmesan cheese and a sprinkle of Savory Sunny Seed Mix, if desired.

Serves 4. Preparation time: 20 minutes.

Nutrition Facts

	calories	total fat	carbs	protein
Mixed Type:	266	14g	29g	13g
Carb Type:	206	9g	28g	9g
Protein Type:	388	22g	25g	26g

Cooking Tips

PT: Can add 2 cups leftover meats or fish at the last minute or make sure you serve some meat protein with the meal. Substitute some asparagus, green beans, cauliflower and vegetables recommended for your type.

CT: Reduce or eliminate the cheese. You can add broken "Vegetable Crispers" or reduce seed mix to 1 tsp per serving.

Notes and Suggestions

Spaghetti squash makes a nice substitute for pasta. Zucchini or summer squash can also be made into noodles by shaving off long, thin, wide strips with a vegetable peeler. Or create authentic long thin spaghetti or angel hair shape by putting the squash through a special "Spiral Slicer" gadget. See Recommended Ingredients Section (page 249) and Zucchetti Pasta recipe (page 234) in Raw, Sprouted and Fermented chapter.

Basic Stuffed Eggs

"Deviled" Eggs, the name coined because of the deviled ham often used as an ingredient, is an ominous name for such a heavenly food.

6	large organic eggs
1/3	cup Basic Mayonnaise (page 238)
2	tsp Dijon or your favorite mustard
1/2	tsp Spike or Mrs. Dash vegetable seasoning
2–3	grinds freshly ground black pepper
	paprika and dill for garnish

Nutrition Facts

calories	total fat	carbs	protein
77	5g	1g	6g

Cooking Tips

PT: Opt for some of the high purine meat fillings like anchovies or herring, dark meat turkey ham, etc.

CT: Lean toward including more of the lower fat vegetable, herb and condiment ingredients.

Notes and Suggestions

Deviled or Stuffed Eggs remain a classic today, open to the addition of anything from ham to caviar. These old favorites can be simple or elegant, but offer a host of opportunities for healthier ingredients. They are great snacks. Use them as the protein component for a meal, combined with some fresh vegetables—especially for a CT—either on a large salad platter, or with spring or summer green salads. They could also add interest to a Spinach Salad for MX or PT, but opt for incorporating some additional meat or fish protein like turkey ham or bacon, anchovies, or caviar into the fillings or the meal.

more variations

Vegetables or Herbs

add 1–2 Tbsp fresh chopped parsley, scallion, dill, marjoram, basil, lemon basil, lemon balm, or even lavender.

Anchovies

add 2 oz finely chopped anchovies.

Vegetable Essences

drizzle tops of stuffed eggs with tiny splashes of Vegetable Essences from squeeze bottle (page 247).

1 boil water in a medium saucepan over high heat. Add eggs, return to boiling and reduce heat to simmer. Cook lightly, 5–6 minutes. Pour off hot water and replace with cold water to cool eggs.

2 when cool enough to handle, peel eggs and cut in half lengthwise. Remove egg yolks to small bowl. Place white halves on serving or dinner plate.

3 mash yolks with fork until smooth. If they are hardcooked, you can push them through a fine sieve, but don't use a food processor, as they will become gummy. Add mayonnaise, mustard, salt and pepper. Whisk briefly to blend and fluff mixture. Add any desired fillings at this point.

4 fill the egg halves with a teaspoon, mounding the fluffy yolk mixture decoratively. Sprinkle every other stuffed egg with dillweed or paprika. Serve right away or cover and refrigerate.

Serves 6. Preparation time: 20 minutes.

variations

Classic Devils

add 2 Tbsp finely chopped turkey ham and 1 more tsp mustard.

Remoulade

use Dijon Remoulade (page 238) instead of mayo.

Smoked Salmon and Crème Fraîche

substitute crème fraîche for mayonnaise and add about 2 Tbsp finely chopped smoked salmon or lox.

Green or Black Olives

add 1 Tbsp chopped black or green pimento-stuffed olives.

Caviar

use crème fraîche or sour cream instead of mayo. Stir in 1 heaping Tbsp black or red caviar. Or alternate eggs with a tiny dollop of each.

Crustless Quiche

This amazing quiche makes its own crust, updated here with a little low-carb, no-grain magic.

2	tsp organic butter or coconut oil
1/2	small red onion, cut in slivers
2	cups broccoli flowerettes
1/4	cup chopped parsley
2	tsp dried basil
4	med whole eggs
1/2	cup whole milk
1/4	cup Beans 'R' Us bean flour, full-fat or soy flour (page 252)
1	Tbsp Dijon mustard
	salt and pepper
1/3	cup raw, organic cheese of choice, shredded

1 preheat oven to 350°F.

2 sauté red onion and broccoli in butter in skillet over medium heat. Add chopped parsley and basil and stir to combine. Turn off heat.

3 beat eggs in bowl with milk, flour, Dijon mustard, salt and pepper. Place in small, greased casserole. Top with cheese. Bake for 15–18 minutes, until set.

4 remove from oven, cut in wedges and serve.

Serves 4. Preparation time: 30 minutes.

Nutrition Facts

	calories	total fat	carbs	protein
Mixed Type:	180	11g	8g	12g
Carb Type:	153	9g	8g	10g
Protein Type:	215	14g	8g	14g

Cooking Tips

PT: Add 4 strips turkey bacon, or 1/2 cup leftover turkey or salmon.

CT: Reduce cheese to 2 Tbsp shredded, low-fat Parmesan or Romano sprinkled on top.

Notes and Suggestions

This egg dish would be nice served as a main entrée for brunch or supper with Spinach Salad or Middle Eastern Salad.

Egg Foo Yung

This inspiration from the Orient is a novel way to incorporate bits of leftover vegetables and meats.

1	Tbsp plus 1 tsp melted butter or coconut oil
1	tsp roasted sesame oil
2	slices fresh ginger root, scraped and minced
2	med scallions or green onions, chopped
2/3	cup sliced mushrooms
1	cup mung bean sprouts
4	large eggs
2	tsp tamari soy sauce
1	Tbsp arrowroot or Beans 'R' Us flour (page 252)
1/2	cup spiced tea or Chai tea (optional)
1/2	cup mushroom soup (optional)
1/2	cup clean, filtered water

Nutrition Facts

	calories	total fat	carbs	protein
Mixed Type:	176	11g	11g	8g
Carb Type:	155	9g	12g	8g
Protein Type:	201	2g	12g	12g

Cooking Tips

PT: Increase mushrooms to 1 cup. Add 1/3 cup chopped, leftover turkey ham, beef, or cooked, dark meat chicken after vegetables are cooked.

CT: Reduce butter or oil to 2 tsp, using paper towel to brush on skillet. Optional variation: Instead of mushrooms, add 1/3 cup each finely chopped red pepper and broccoli with the scallions. Stir in 1/4 cup chopped parsley at the end.

Notes and Suggestions

These flat egg pancakes are easier and faster to make than a large omelet. Besides being a good way to incorporate lots of fresh, healthy ingredients, they are a clever wrap or base for fillings—even cold, spread with mayo, fresh spinach and sliced tomato. Tote leftovers filled with sprouts and spreads for "sandwiches." While eggs are considered a quality protein, PT's should also incorporate some meat.

1 combine melted butter and sesame oil in custard cup. Add about 2 tsp to a large skillet heated on medium high. Add ginger root and stir.

2 add scallions and mushrooms. Sauté for 1 minute. Then add bean sprouts and snow peas and continue cooking until mushrooms soften and sprouts start to wilt, 1–2 minutes. Remove from heat and transfer to mixing bowl.

3 into small bowl, break eggs. Add soy sauce and arrowroot, whisking with a wire whisk to blend. Pour egg mixture over vegetables in large bowl.

4 return skillet to fire. Coat skillet with a little more oil mixture and scoop veggie-egg batter, 1/4 cup at a time, into mounds in skillet. Cook for 2–3 minutes, until brown on one side, then turn over carefully with spatula. When moisture has congealed, remove pancakes to serving platter.

5 if sauce is desired, thin 1/2 cup organic mushroom soup with water and heat slightly. For more of a "sweet 'n spicy" sauce, mix 1 Tbsp arrowroot or bean flour with 1/2 cup spiced or Chai tea and 1/2 cup water in small saucepan. Bring to a boil and stir until thickened. Use 1 Tbsp per two egg foo yung servings.

Serves 4. Preparation time: 15 minutes.

Egg Salad with Artichokes

Classic egg salad becomes elevated to another level with the addition of quartered artichoke hearts.

4	eggs, semi-hardcooked (about 5 minutes)
1	14 oz can artichoke hearts, drained and quartered
1	med scallion or green onion, white part, chopped
1/3	cup Basic Mayonnaise or Dijon Remoulade (page 238)
2	chopped anchovy filets or anchovy paste, if desired
1	tsp capers, drained, if desired

1 peel and chop eggs in mixing bowl. Add quartered artichoke hearts, green onions, and basic mayonnaise or Dijon Remoulade, and stir to combine.

2 top with chopped anchovies or drizzle with anchovy paste and 1 tsp capers, optional. Serve immediately if ingredients are already cold, or refrigerate for 10–15 minutes.

Serves 4. Preparation time: 10 minutes.

Nutrition Facts

	calories	total fat	carbs	protein
Mixed Type:	114	6g	5g	9g
Carb Type:	100	4g	7g	8g
Protein Type:	118	6g	5g	10g

Cooking Tips

PT: Add anchovies or serve with additional meat protein.

CT: Omit anchovies. Reduce mayonnaise to 3 Tbsp. Alternately, use half basic mayo and half lowfat yogurt.

Notes and Suggestions

This could be a heavenly filling for a Roll-Up, or an accompaniment for Grecian Spinach for a PT, along with some more concentrated protein. Or serve as a main salad for a CT lunch. It is truly delicious and different.

Eggs Benedict Florentine

Enjoy this version of the classic egg dish on a bed of seasoned spinach for an easy, but upscale luncheon or stay-at-home Sunday brunch with the family.

Spinach

1	tsp organic butter or coconut oil
3	med scallions, sliced
6	oz turkey ham or turkey bacon
2	10 oz bags baby spinach

Hollandaise

2	Tbsp organic butter
1½	tsp fresh lemon, juice
1	large whole egg, divided
½	tsp water

Eggs and Assembly

4	large eggs

Nutrition Facts

	calories	total fat	carbs	protein
Mixed Type:	251	16g	8g	20g
Carb Type:	188	14g	2g	13g
Protein Type:	268	17g	8g	22g

Cooking Tips

PT: This is an ideal dish for PT, with a good balance of egg and meat protein, and spinach, which is an excellent vegetable for you. Increase meat to 8 oz.

CT: Reduce meat to 4 oz. Reduce the Hollandaise sauce to 1 tsp per serving, drizzled over the eggs.

Spinach

1 preheat oven to 375°F. In large skillet or ovenproof ceramic casserole over medium high, sauté scallions in butter for 1–2 minutes. Add chopped turkey ham or bacon and sauté 2 or 3 minutes longer, until meat starts to crisp and/or brown.

2 add spinach to pan and stir-sauté until it starts to wilt. Season with salt and pepper. Remove from heat. Transfer spinach to pie plate or ovenware, if applicable. Cover and place in oven.

Hollandaise

1 melt butter with lemon in small saucepan over medium low heat. Separate the egg, saving white to add to the 4 whole eggs.

2 beat egg yolk with ½ tsp water, just to blend in small cup or custard cup. Stir in a little of the hot butter, stirring with a wire whisk to blend and "temper" or elevate temperature of egg yolks. Blend yolks, stirring constantly, with the rest of the lemon butter to make a smooth sauce. Put pan off and on burner, three or four times, to avoid overcooking. When thick, remove from heat.

Eggs and Assembly

1 take casserole with spinach out of oven. Remove cover and break four eggs over top of spinach, making little nests or indentations for eggs to rest, if necessary. Add the remaining egg white.

2 replace cover and return to oven for 4–5 minutes, just until whites start to firm. Remove from oven, remove cover and pour or spoon warm hollandaise over top of eggs. Replace cover.

Serves 4. Preparation time: 15 minutes.

Vegetable Frittata

A frittata is like an omelet with no flipping and a quiche with no crust—a fast egg dish that can be made with a variety of vegetables, meats and cheeses.

2	Tbsp organic butter or coconut oil
3/4	cup chopped red onion
1	lb mushrooms or red peppers, sliced
4	cups chopped broccoli, cauliflower, zucchinis, artichoke hearts, asparagus, spinach, or other dark greens
2	Tbsp fresh marjoram
8	med eggs
1/4	cup whole or lowfat milk
2	tsp dry mustard or 2 tsp prepared mustard
1	tsp freshly ground black pepper
2	tsp Spike vegetable seasoning or Mrs. Dash
2	tsp Parsley Vegetable Essence (page 247)

1 heat oil in large skillet over medium heat. Add onions and mushrooms, stirring until onions are translucent, 1–2 minutes.

2 add chopped vegetables and marjoram leaves. Stir-sauté until vegetables start to turn bright green or soften. Reduce heat to medium or medium low.

3 break 8 eggs into small bowl. Add milk, dry or prepared mustard, and pepper. Use a fork just to break up yolks, so mixture looks marbleized. Pour over vegetables in skillet.

4 sprinkle all over with Spike. Cook 3–4 minutes, just until eggs start to set. Remove from heat and decorate top with a few drizzles of Parsley Vegetable Essence.

Serves 4. Preparation time: 15 minutes.

Nutrition Facts

	calories	total fat	carbs	protein
Mixed Type:	288	18g	15g	20g
Carb Type:	222	14g	9g	16g
Protein Type:	310	21g	11g	22g

Cooking Tips

PT: Sauté 4 strips chopped turkey bacon in skillet first, then add only 1/2 cup onions. Can increase mushrooms to 1 1/2 lb. Choose spinach for the greens.

CT: Reduce oil to 1 Tbsp. Use lowfat milk.

Notes and Suggestions

This is another one of those recipes with an endless array of possibilities. A good quick meal for using up what you have on hand. Don't overcook the eggs.

Vegetable Quiche

Quiche is a classic French egg presentation, with almost limitless possibilities for incorporating high-quality, healthy ingredients.

Crust

1/2	cup organic flax seeds, ground in coffee grinder or blender
1/2	cup organic sesame seeds, ground
1	Tbsp raw or organic butter, cold
1/2	cup Swiss or cheddar cheese, grated
3/4	tsp allspice
1/2	tsp Spike vegetable seasoning or Mrs. Dash

Filling

2	tsp coconut oil
6	slices turkey bacon, chopped
1/3	cup red onion, chopped
2	cups broccoli, broccoli rabe or cauliflower, chopped
2	tsp dried basil

Custard

4	med eggs
1/2	cup whole milk
3/4	tsp nutmeg
1	tsp salt
1/2	tsp pepper

Nutrition Facts

	calories	total fat	carbs	protein
Mixed Type:	292	22g	12g	14g
Carb Type:	292	22g	12g	14g
Protein Type:	304	22g	12g	17g

Cooking Tips

PT: Instead of turkey bacon, 1/2 cup left-over cooked meats or salmon can be used as a variation.

CT: Follow recipe as is.

Notes and Suggestions

Another classic vehicle for adding vegetables of all kinds. Seasoned with herbs, spinach or broccoli, this dish creates a good camouflage for Swiss chard, beet greens, kale, some of those "less popular" vegetables. Note: at times broccoli rabe can be somewhat bitter tasting, but is very healthy.

Crust

1 Preheat oven to 370°F. In food processor workbowl, add ground flax, ground sesame seed, cold butter, shredded cheese, allspice and Spike. Pulse for 5 seconds, only until mixture starts to come together. Do not overprocess.

2 pat mixture evenly into lightly greased, 8" shallow pie pan.

Filling

1 heat medium skillet on medium high heat. Add coconut oil, a layer of turkey bacon and onions, broccoli, sautéing for 3–5 minutes until onions turn translucent and broccoli color brightens. Sprinkle with basil, remove from heat, and pile into crust.

Custard

1 break eggs into bowl, add milk, nutmeg, salt and pepper and stir with a fork to blend. Pour over vegetable or vegetable/meat filling.

2 bake in preheated 375° oven for 12–15 minutes, only until crust is getting brown and eggs have started to set. Middle will still be slightly soft.

Serves 6. Preparation time: 20 minutes.

Baked Herbed Salmon

A traditional Mediterranean herb sauce for an elegant fish dinner that's fast, tasty and low carb. The fish bakes with the sauce, while the rest of the meal is prepared.

4	6 oz wild Alaskan Salmon filets (page 251)
1	Tbsp extra virgin olive oil
2	med garlic cloves
½	tsp Spike vegetable seasoning or Mrs. Dash
1	tsp ground cumin seed
½	tsp black pepper
1	Tbsp capers or green olives
1	cup flat-leaf Italian parsley
1	cup cilantro leaves
2	tsp grated lemon rind or 3-4 drops lemon oil
⅓	cup fresh lemon juice

1 preheat oven to 350°F. Rinse fish and place on lightly greased cookie sheet or ceramic casserole. Sprinkle fish with salt and pepper.

2 in food processor, make marinade/sauce by combining olive oil, garlic, Spike, cumin, pepper, capers, parsley, cilantro, lemon rind or oil, and lemon juice.

3 spread over fish in pan. Bake for 13–15 minutes, or until fish flakes easily with fork.

Serves 4. Preparation time: 10 minutes.

Nutrition Facts

calories	total fat	carbs	protein
291	14g	4g	35g

Cooking Tips

PT: Follow as is.

CT: Salmon is a higher fat fish, not recommended for your type. Prepare this recipe with another fish, such as tilapia.

Notes and Suggestions

Combine this entrée with a healthy portion of a vegetable salad such as Mediterranean Salad or Chop Chop Garden Salad for a menu. If you find that this isn't enough food for you, you don't feel quite satisfied, or just plain need more, add a vegetable side dish such as leftover Green Bean Casserole or a serving of Mushroom Cream Soup.

Broiled Lemon Salmon

Fresh lemon juice is the key to making broiled salmon exceptional.

1	Tbsp tamari soy sauce
1	garlic clove, minced
1/3	cup fresh lemon juice
1	tsp extra virgin olive oil
2	Tbsp chopped chives
4	6 oz wild, red Alaskan salmon filets (page 251)
1	whole lemon, cut into 1/8" slices

Nutrition Facts

calories	total fat	carbs	protein
271	11g	4g	37g

Cooking Tips

PT: An ideal dish for you.

CT: This is not a good dish for your type, since salmon is not a recommended fish. Prepare with another fish like tilapia, which is relatively low in mercury.

Notes and Suggestions

Serve this simple-to-make dish with Grecian Spinach or Broccoli-in-a-Hurry Curry.

1 mix tamari, garlic, lemon juice, olive oil, and chives together.

2 place salmon filets in flat pan. Cover with marinade and lemon slices. Marinate, turning occasionally, for 20–30 minutes. Remove lemon slices from fish and place around pan.

3 broil salmon with rack set 6" under broiler unit for 3–4 minutes. Turn salmon carefully and continue to broil another 3 minutes, or until brown and fish flakes easily.

4 remove to serving platter. Place lemon slices on top of fish. Pour any remaining marinade over. Serve immediately.

Serves 4. Preparation time: 10 minutes.

Miso Glazed Salmon

The fermented Japanese soybean paste called miso is a high-flavor, low-carb ingredient for adding heartiness, deep color and healthy nutrition to foods.

2	Tbsp miso, soybean paste
2	Tbsp low sodium tamari soy sauce
2	Tbsp apple cider or juice
2	tsp grated ginger root
½	tsp ground allspice or nutmeg
	dash vegetable oil for greasing pan
4	6 oz wild, red Alaskan salmon filets, cut in half (page 251)
1	Tbsp chopped fresh chives

1 preheat broiler. In small bowl, whisk soybean paste with tamari, apple juice, ginger, allspice, and 1 Tbsp water.

2 place salmon fillets in a shallow baking pan rubbed lightly with oil. Spoon miso mixture evenly over salmon.

3 broil 8–10 minutes, basting two or more times with marinade, until fish flakes with a fork. Do not overcook.

4 remove to serving platter. Sprinkle with chopped chives.

Serves 4. Preparation time: 15 minutes.

Nutrition Facts

	calories	total fat	carbs	protein
Mixed Type:	286	12g	4g	39g
Protein Type:	382	16g	6g	52g

Cooking Tips

PT: This dish is a good one for you, with a larger portion, so serve 3.

CT: Salmon is too high fat a fish for you. Substitute with tilapia.

Notes and Suggestions

This fast and easy salmon dish could be a lifesaver after a busy day. Pair it with a Hot and Sour Soup, Sea Side Salad, or simply some fast Braised Brazilian Greens for a speedy supper. Miso is one of the healthier forms of soy, a salty, fermented, soybean paste that is available in Oriental or natural foods section and keeps indefinitely in your refrigerator.

Nouveau Salmon Nicoise

This colorful arranged salad comes from Nice, on the French Riviera. But you can substitute your own similar favorite vegetables, the "best" foods for your own taste and eating plan.

1	can wild, red Alaskan salmon, drained and chunked (page 251)
2	quarts romaine lettuce leaves, torn
1	cup artichoke hearts, drained and quartered
8	black and green olives
¾	cup jicama, peeled and cut into matchsticks
1	cup clover or broccoli sprouts
¼	cup pepperoncini peppers
4	anchovy filets
½	med avocado, peeled and cut into cubes
⅓	cup Dijon Remoulade Sauce Or Caesar salad dressing (page 238) lemon wedges, garnish

1 arrange lettuce on large serving platter. Arrange mounds of the colorful ingredients over the platter. Spritz with a splash of lemon juice.

2 serve immediately with a small bowl of Dijon Remoulade Sauce or Caesar dressing.

Serves 4. Preparation time: 10 minutes.

Nutrition Facts

	calories	*total fat*	*carbs*	*protein*
Mixed Type:	396	27g	17g	26g
Protein Type:	463	33g	17g	28g

Cooking Tips

PT: Can substitute at least half spinach for romaine and add semi-hardcooked egg halves to the plate. Have more olives.

CT: Not your recommended fish, substitute tilapia for salmon. Omit anchovies. Substitute 2 tsp capers per serving for olives. Use ¼ cup dressing and ¼ cup lowfat yogurt. Use only ½ avocado.

Notes and Suggestions

This is a delicious, versatile meal salad for all types, varying the amount of protein and specific vegetables for your type. PT's, this is an excellent recipe, traditionally calling for those high purine proteins, like anchovies, your metabolic type needs.

Poached Salmon Dijonnaise

Looks and sounds like a gourmet dish, but this simple poached fish is actually fast and easy to prepare.

¼	cup lemon juice or white wine vinegar
1	tsp sea salt or Spike vegetable seasoning
4	wild, red Alaskan salmon filets (page 251)
⅓	cup Dijonnaise (page 238)

1 pour 3 fingers of water, lemon juice, and salt into large, deep ceramic casserole or fish poacher and bring to boil. Reduce heat to simmer.

2 rinse off salmon. Sprinkle with Spike. Slip filets into simmering water and steam gently for 5–8 minutes.

3 remove to serving dish or platter. Serve topped with or accompanied by Dijonnaise Sauce.

Serves 4. Preparation time: 10 minutes.

Nutrition Facts

	calories	*total fat*	*carbs*	*protein*
Mixed Type:	372	23g	2g	38g
Carb Type:	196	10g	4g	14g
Protein Type:	432	30g	2g	38g

Cooking Tips

PT: This is a good dish for your type.

CT: Substitute tilapia for salmon.

Notes and Suggestions

A suggestion for making this easy, but sophisticated, recipe part of a whole menu is to serve it with Roasted Asparagus or Cauliflower with Tapenade Crown. If you're a CT, try it with a steamed vegetable like broccoli and zucchini, or Brussels Sprout Trio.

Roasted Salmon with Pesto Crust

Quick, easy and sinfully delicious, this elegant recipe is the fruit of those batch cooking sessions you wisely scheduled, producing the wonderful pesto that's right in your fridge.

6	wild red Alaskan salmon filets, rinsed and patted dry (page 251)
1/2	cup Basil Pesto (page 239)
1	Tbsp plus 1 tsp coconut oil
1	small shallot or 2 small green onions, minced
2	10 oz pkgs baby spinach leaves, washed
	sea salt and freshly ground black pepper
6	cherry tomatoes (optional) or
6	Tbsp Red Onion Cilantro Relish, optional (page 245)

Nutrition Facts

	calories	total fat	carbs	protein
Mixed Type:	338	18g	16g	30g
Carb Type:	330	22g	18g	18g
Protein Type:	368	18g	20g	30g

Cooking Tips

PT: Use 2/3 cup Red Onion Relish.

CT: Salmon is not a recommended fish, so substitute another kind like tilapia. You could substitute another dark leafy green such as bok choy for variety.

Notes and Suggestions

This could be considered a meal in itself, since the vegetable is included. But you might want to accompany it with a mixed green salad, topped with crunchy herbed sprouts and some additional salad dressing.

1 preheat oven to 400°F. Spread 2 Tbsp pesto over salmon filets.

2 in ovenproof skillet over high heat, melt 2 tsp of the coconut oil. Sear the salmon, pesto side down, 2–3 minutes. Gently turn over filets with long spatula. Place in oven for 5–6 minutes until lightly cooked through.

3 add remaining oil and minced shallot to another skillet, stirring until onion is translucent, about 1 minute. Squeeze out any extra moisture from spinach leaves and pat dry. Add with salt and pepper to skillet and sauté quickly over high heat, about 1–2 minutes.

4 divide spinach onto serving plates as a bed for salmon. Place a salmon filet on top. Garnish with 1–2 cherry tomatoes or Red Onion Cilantro Relish.

Serves 6. Preparation time: 15 minutes.

Salmon Crêpes

This upscale but easy entrée folds a vegetable-fish filling into No-Grain Crêpes for a special meal from foods you may already have in your pantry.

8	No-Grain Crêpes (See page 203)
1	Tbsp organic butter or coconut oil
1	med shallot or 2 garlic cloves, minced
1	10 oz pkg fresh spinach
2	cups fresh or canned asparagus, chopped
1	can artichoke hearts, drained and quartered
1	tsp Braggs Liquid Amino's or Spike vegetable seasoning
1	14 oz can wild, red Alaskan salmon, drained (page 251)
4	Tbsp Remoulade Sauce (page 238)

1 prepare crêpes or pull already-prepared portions from your freezer. If crêpes are frozen, moisten slightly with water or brush lightly with oil. Preheat oven to 350°F.

2 in medium skillet over medium low, melt butter and sauté minced shallot or garlic until translucent. If using fresh asparagus, add it at this point and sauté until it starts to brighten. If using canned or frozen asparagus, add it with the artichokes.

3 add spinach leaves and sauté until spinach starts to wilt. Add remaining vegetables and sprinkle with Bragg's or Spike. Add drained canned salmon chunks and heat through.

4 divide mixture among 8 crêpes. Place about $1/4$ cup filling on each crêpe, topping with a 2 tsp portion to start of Remoulade Sauce before rolling up. Place filled crêpes, edges down, in lightly buttered ceramic or glass casserole. Place in preheated oven for approximately 5–6 minutes, until heated through.

5 remove from oven to hot pad on table. Serve immediately, two crêpes per serving.

Serves 4. Preparation time: 15 minutes.

Nutrition Facts

	calories	total fat	carbs	protein
Mixed Type:	523	31g	34g	32g
Carb Type:	393	27g	23g	18g
Protein Type:	546	34g	34g	32g

Cooking Tips

PT: An ideal PT type dish. You could also make this with lox or smoked salmon, about 10 oz.

CT: This dish is not well suited to your type with these ingredients. However, you could substitute another fish such as tilapia or even light meat chicken, or use 3 semi-hardcooked eggs. Replace the vegetables with dark greens and others more suited to your type.

Notes and Suggestions

This entrée has both protein and vegetables, but you may find that you want to add a green salad with sprouts and Sunny Seed Salad Dressing or a vegetable side. If this is not enough to make you PT's feel satisfied, trying increasing the protein in the dish. Or use 2 Tbsp Remoulade Sauce per serving. Again, these are to be considered suggestions or starting points for modifying recipes and meals to achieve your optimum balance. Many of the recipes represent minimums, so listen to your body and see what works for you.

Salmon Seviche

In South America, Japan, and other regions, seviche or ceviche is served as a marinated raw fish appetizer. It is another popular way to preserve flavor, nutrition, and digestibility of fresh seafood.

1	lb fresh, wild red Alaskan salmon (page 251)
⅓	cup red onion, finely diced
1	cup fresh lime juice
2	Tbsp seeded serrano pepper, finely chopped or
1	chili pepper, smashed
2	tsp sea salt
1	cup chopped tomatoes
2	cups chopped cilantro or parsley

Nutrition Facts

	calories	total fat	carbs	protein
Mixed Type:	205	7g	10g	26g
Carb Type:	197	12g	10g	14g
Protein Type:	238	10g	11g	26g

Cooking Tips

PT: A good summer dish for you, but reduce the tomatoes to ½ cup and add ½ cup finely chopped celery.

CT: Salmon is not a recommended fish for your type: substitute tilapia for salmon.

Notes and Suggestions

This adaptation of the South American favorite raw fish salad is traditionally made with other high purine fish like mussels or clams. It is often served as an appetizer, but could become the main protein in a meal salad platter like Nouveau Salmon Nicoise or a light summer antipasto.

1 skin fish and chop into ¼–½" pieces. Combine salmon, chopped red onion, lime juice, pepper, and salt. Marinate for several hours or overnight.

2 ten to fifteen minutes before serving, add chopped tomatoes and cilantro and/or parsley, and stir to combine. Serve accompanied by butter lettuce or other leafy salad greens.

Serves 4. Preparation time: 10 minutes.

THE RECIPES: Juices & Smoothies

The most nutritious way to eat your veggies is though juicing. Juicing raw vegetables concentrates the valuable nutrients, enzymes and energy, the essence of the plant, into powerful doses of healing nutrition in a glass.

All live plant foods can be made into juice. However, vegetable juices are preferred above all, because of their superior nutritive, healing and tonic effect. The valuable anti-oxidants and enzymes in live foods are altered and destroyed by heat and cooking. Juicing protects the live, biochemically active factors in enzymes, which are most beneficial for their repair, cleansing and detoxifying functions in the body. Fruit juices are cleansing, but also contain highly concentrated simple sugars that can lift the blood sugar too rapidly, causing excessive insulin production. Carrots and other high-glycemic or sugar vegetables can have the same effect, so I recommend that they be minimized. Keeping the blood sugar stable and steady is one of the top goals of the Total Health Program.

The best juices nutritionally are the green juices: kale, chard, dandelion greens, spinach, turnip and mustard greens, parsley, and fresh herbs. These green juices contain the valuable nutrient, chlorophyll, which oxygenates and purifies the blood and tissues. While some of these lower-on-the-popularity-poll juices are strong in flavor, small amounts of ginger, garlic or herbs can be added to "sweeten" the slightly bitter taste of some of them. Another way to achieve this and improve the appearance is to "float" small quantities of various colored, flavored juices on top of the greens. Other ways to bolster the nutritional and health benefits are to juice sprouts and to add small amounts of concentrated foods like chlorella, mint, and high omega-3 oils such as fish and cod liver oil.

Regardless of the fact that they are commonly mixed today, it is best to keep vegetable and fruit juices separate. The fibrous pulp of fruits and vegetable juice is definitely valuable, as the non-absorbable complex carbohydrates it contains help to keep blood sugar stabilized. Fibers or pulps can be added back for added bulk and structure to non-grain recipes, including baked goods. The preferred juice extractor for creating valuable live juices is the Omega 8002, discussed in the "Recommended Ingredients and Products Locator" in the Appendix page 249.

It is highly recommended to use the preferred and recommended vegetables for your metabolic type as discussed in Chapter 5, mixing and matching as you choose. Any combinations of your recommended vegetables are okay. You will soon discover the joys and delights of consuming fresh juice on a regular, daily basis, something your body will tell you is ideal for lifting your energy and your spirits.

Almond Nut Milk

A smart substitute for dairy, this smooth beverage can be easily made in your own blender.

1	cup raw almonds
4	cups cold, clean filtered water
½	tsp vanilla extract

1 add almonds through hole in top of blender while machine is running. Process until nuts become mealy.

2 slowly start to add a small amount of water. As mixture blends and almonds go into suspension, add remaining water and vanilla extract. Blend until light, creamy and frothy.

Serves 4. Serving size: About 1 cup. Preparation time: 5 minutes.

Nutrition Facts

	calories	*total fat*	*carbs*	*protein*
unstrained	208	18g	7g	8g
strained	104	9g	4g	4g

Cooking Tips

Normally it isn't critical to strain the drink, especially because you lose some of the valuable nut meal. But if you're serving this for guests, you can strain it through a sieve, which removes the solids, reduces the granular texture and reduces fat, protein and calorie content of the milk.

You can also create "blanched, skinned" almonds by pouring hot water over raw almonds and letting them set till the water gets tepid. The skins slip off easily by squeezing nut between thumb and forefinger into a jar. (See detailed description in Zucchini Muffins, page 210.)

Notes and Suggestions

This non-dairy milk can be enjoyed as is, or to replace dairy milk in shakes, smoothies, soups and other applications. Raw almonds are naturally sweet, but if you still haven't kicked your super sweet-tooth addiction you can blend this with Stevia sweetener for more sweetness. This milk can also be made with other raw (preferably organic) nuts.

Soaking and sprouting the almonds (and any raw nuts and seeds) significantly increases their digestibility. Cover with clean water in a glass jar, soak overnight, then drain off the soak water. They won't have long "tails," but letting the soaked, drained nuts sprout, even for 3 hours, increases the bioavailability of nutrients to your body.

Breakfast Slurpy Pudding

This is a quick and thick blender concoction for a fast breakfast. It's made like a shake, but thick like a pudding, due to the thickening power of the flax and psyllium. Super fiber load.

1/3	cup soaked, organic almonds
2	Tbsp organic flax seeds
3	Tbsp shredded coconut
1	Tbsp psyllium seed husks (page 252)
1/2	tsp cardamom pods
2	cups brewed herbal tea
1	cup clean, filtered water
1/4	(1 oz) banana Or
1	Tbsp blueberry or cherry juice concentrate

Nutrition Facts

calories	total fat	carbs	protein
266	18g	21g	9g

1 in blender or food processor fitted with steel blade, grind soaked almonds, flax seed, coconut, psyllium seed, and cardamom pods until coarsely ground.

2 slowly add brewed tea and water. Process until smooth.

3 add banana or fruit concentrate. Process until mixture becomes thick.

4 spoon into large glass or bowl. Eat with a spoon right away.

Serves 2. Serving Size: 1³/4 cup per serving. Preparation time: 5 minutes.

Cheery Egg Nog

The traditional holiday cup of cheer with healthy, high-quality ingredients.

4	whole eggs
1	cup raw cream
3	cups whole raw milk
2	tsp vanilla
2	tsp ground nutmeg or cinnamon
¼	cup apple juice concentrate Or
3	Tbsp blueberry or cherry juice concentrate

Nutrition Facts

calories	total fat	carbs	protein
356	20g	28g	15g

1 into blender container add cream, milk, vanilla, nutmeg and fruit concentrate. Blend on high until creamy and frothy.

2 add raw eggs and pulse a few times until just blended and creamy. Serve immediately, sprinkled with nutmeg or cinnamon.

Serves 4. Serving size: About 1 cup. Preparation time: 5 minutes.

Nut Shake Too

This even faster version of a smoothie or shake can be a lifesaver when you need to eat, but don't even have time to think. Recommendation: Breathe while blending.

1	Tbsp raw nut butter (almond, sesame, macadamia, walnut, pecan,etc.)
2	Tbsp dry, unsweetened coconut
2	cups clean, filtered cold water
½	packet SteviaPlus, alternative sweetener (page 253)
1	whole egg

Nutrition Facts

calories	total fat	carbs	protein
290	23g	7g	12g

1 in blender container, process nut butter, coconut, water, and SteviaPlus. Process on high until smooth and frothy. Add whole egg and pulse briefly to blend.

2 pour into glass and enjoy.

Serves 1.Serving size: 2 cup serving. Preparation time: 5 minutes.

Pineapple Elixir

For a special occasion or holiday treat, indulge yourself with this sumptuous beverage.

³⁄4	cup freshly squeezed pineapple juice
2	cups mint tea
1″	piece fresh ginger root, scraped with spoon
1–2	drops mint extract, optional

1 in blender container, combine pineapple juice and mint tea.

2 throw in chopped ginger root and mint extract, if desired. Blend on high.

3 strain and serve immediately.

Serves 2. Serving size: generous 1¹⁄3 cup. Preparation time: 5 minutes.

Nutrition Facts

calories	total fat	carbs	protein
58	0g	14g	0g

Cooking Tips

Though healthy, even fresh fruit juice is concentrated simple sugars, so enjoy only occasionally. If you feel tired, hungry or shaky immediately or within 2 hours of drinking, this is a sign that the carbohydrates are upsetting your blood sugar balance. You can minimize this somewhat by adding protein, such as blending nut butter with the juice or drinking it with a meal or snack.

Notes and Suggestions

You can substitute other fresh squeezed juices, even vegetable juices, in this beverage. See page 206 for what to do with your leftover pineapple pulp.

Sprouted Seed Shake

Another fast and healthy version of a quick smoothie for breakfast or snack.

½	cup sprouted Basic Sunny Seed Mix (page 215)
1	slice ginger root
1	Tbsp blueberry or cherry juice concentrate
2	cups clean, filtered water
¼	tsp (½ pkt) SteviaPlus alternative sweetener (page 253)

1 soak ¼ cup Basic Sunny Seed Mix overnight in clean, filtered water. Drain off soak water. Or even better, measure out ½ cup soaked seeds that have been allowed to sprout.

2 place soaked/sprouted seeds, ginger and fruit concentrate in blender container. Turn on blender and start to add water, gradually at first, to allow seeds to chop and blend.

3 add remaining water and alternative sweetener. Blend on high until drink is smooth and frothy. Drink immediately.

Serves 1. Preparation time: 5 minutes.

Nutrition Facts

calories	total fat	carbs	protein
303	23g	17g	11g

Cooking Tips

You might want to strain this through a fine sieve before drinking. CT's will want to watch the amount of seeds they consume, but sprouting reduces the carbs and makes them more digestible for you, as well. See Sprouting in Raw, Sprouted & Fermented Foods chapter (page 225).

Notes and Suggestions

Sprouting increases the nutrition and digestibility of nuts and seeds, so anytime you can sprout before using means you get more nutritional bonus points. Even simply soaking the seeds overnight makes them more digestible, so consider getting into the habit of this.

Sunny Almond Shake

This fix-it-fast nut shake is a basic recipe you can vary to nourish yourself for breakfast, snack or on-the-run.

2	Tbsp organic almonds
2	Tbsp organic sunflower seeds
2	Tbsp organic flax seeds
3	cups clean, filtered water (1½ cups if using juice)
½	cup fresh apple cider or pineapple juice Or
½	cup fresh blueberries or raspberries
½	tsp vanilla extract
½	tsp nutmeg

1 process almonds, sunflower, and flax seeds on high in covered blender container, until coarsely ground.

2 pour in water slowly at first, letting blades reduce ingredients to a thick consistency. Add remaining liquid and continue blending.

3 add apple cider, juice or berries, vanilla extract, and nutmeg, and blend until frothy. Pour in glass and drink immediately.

Serves 2. Preparation time: 5 minutes.

Nutrition Facts

calories	total fat	carbs	protein
218	13g	20g	7g

Cooking Tips

PT: A good source of protein, the nuts and seeds can help you make it through the morning, although you probably will want to consume a larger serving.

CT: Watch how frequently you choose to use nuts and seeds, since they are recommended only sparingly for your type due to the fat content.

Notes and Suggestions

Simply soaking the nuts and seeds overnight will do a lot to increase the digestibility and healthfulness of this drink. Be sure to drain off soak liquid and rinse before blending with clean water. This probably won't seem that sweet to you at first. But as you get over your sugar addiction, you will start to appreciate the subtle flavors of the ingredients themselves, and the nourishing feeling that a stable, sustained blood sugar level imparts.

Sweet Sunny Seed Shake

One of those quick recipes when you're really pressed for time. You'll really appreciate the few minutes you took preparing the mix ahead...

2	**Tbsp Sweet Sunny Seed Mix (page 215)**
2	**cups clean, cold, filtered water**
1	**whole egg**

1 add sweet seed mix through small hole in top of blender cover, while machine is running on medium low. Replace top. Process to start breaking up seeds.

2 gradually add about $1/4$ of the water and process for a minute or so until mixture starts to blend. Continue, adding remaining water. Blend on high until shake is smooth and frothy. Stop machine.

3 break raw egg into shake and pulse 1–2 times only to blend. Pour in glass and serve.

Serves 1. Serving size: About 2 cups . Preparation time: 5 minutes.

Nutrition Facts

calories	total fat	carbs	protein
160	14g	6g	8g

Notes and Suggestions

For an even healthier, more digestible variation, simply soak the sweet seed mix overnight, pouring off soak water and rinsing the mix before blending with clean water. Letting the mix "sprout," if you have the time, even for 2–3 hours, really peaks this off the healthiness scale. See Raw, Sprouted & Fermented Foods (page 225).

THE RECIPES: Baked Goods & Desserts

The recipes in this section are designed with a "hint of sweetness." They use small amounts of coconuts, fruits, nuts and flavorings, and very small amounts of natural sweeteners like no-sugar-added fruit concentrates, honey, maple syrup and the non-glycemic, non-synthetic herb Stevia.

The treats in this section are designed to be once-in-awhile indulgences because some are high in calories, so use them sparingly, and only after you have stabilized your metabolism and used EFT to eliminate your cravings. If you find that you start craving more sweets, hold off until you are more in control.

Many of these recipes may not taste very sweet to those used to eating high-sugar foods. But your body will soon learn that not only can it survive without a sugar fix, but your overall health and well-being depends on it. Remember, the more you eat, the more you want. This goes for sugar, salts and fats. Because of the body's highly adaptive character and the addictive nature of sugar, when you reduce or eliminate sugar from your diet in favor of nutrient-dense, lower-carb vegetables and meats, you'll begin to notice that everything tastes sweeter. Regular sweets will begin to seem too sweet. You'll wonder how you ever could have eaten half a dozen chocolate chip cookies at one sitting. And it goes both ways. The more fresh, complex carbohydrate vegetables and high quality foods you eat, the more of them you want. The more stored toxins you get rid of, the more your own body wisdom kicks in and starts craving, at a deep level, the foods that are good for you.

So enjoy these "sweet" recipes. Just go light on this category of foods, and always monitor your reaction after you eat them. Remember, on this eating plan, your LIFE will be sweet!

Cheese Bread

An alternative non-grain bread you can use for sandwiches.

1½	cups deskinned raw almond, macadamia or other nut flour
1	cup Beans 'R' Us bean flour, arrowroot or soy flour (page 252)
1	tsp baking soda
1	tsp ground cumin seed
¼	cup coconut oil, raw or organic butter
1	cup grass-fed sharp cheddar, shredded
3	med eggs, beaten
1	Tbsp honey or
1	packet SteviaPlus alternate sweetener (page 253)

Nutrition Facts

calories	total fat	carbs	protein
323	26g	13g	14g

Cooking Tips

See a more detailed description for making your own nut flour at home, in Zucchini Muffins recipe (page 210). This is a higher fat and protein recipe that would probably satisfy a PT, but wouldn't be as appropriate for someone who is trying to lose weight. Try one of the alternative wraps or Roll-Up suggestions (pages 213–214) instead.

1 preheat oven to 350°F. In mixing bowl, combine nut flour, bean flour, baking soda, and cumin.

2 add coconut oil or butter and shredded cheese and stir until blended.

3 stir in beaten eggs and sweetener. Pour into well greased 4"x 8" loaf pan. Bake until golden brown, approximately 15 minutes.

Serves 9. Preparation time: 10 minutes.

Coconut Custard Flan Pie

This is a rich, custardy dessert made with real coconut milk.

1	recipe Sweet No-Flour Pie Crust (page 202)
2	cups coconut milk
¼	cup raw or organic cream
2	med whole eggs
2	Tbsp maple syrup or 1 pkt SteviaPlus alternative sweetener
1	tsp vanilla extract
1	tsp freshly grated nutmeg

Nutrition Facts

calories	total fat	carbs	protein
338	29g	15g	8g

1 preheat oven to 375°F. In medium bowl or blender container, combine coconut milk, cream, eggs, sweetener, vanilla, and nutmeg. Blend.

2 pour into prepared No-Flour Crust Pie shell. Bake until custard is set and crust sets up, approximately 15–18 minutes. Remove from oven. Place on wire rack to cool slightly.

3 cut into 6–8 servings.

Serves 6. Preparation time: 10 minutes.

Fruit and Nut Torte

An elegant no-grain dessert that will still allow you to stay on your eating plan.

½	cup almonds
2	egg yolks
3	Tbsp maple syrup
2	egg whites
	pinch sea salt
1	recipe Nut Cream (page 235) or Crème Fraîche (page 232)
1	cup fresh blueberries
1	cup fresh raspberries
2	Tbsp blueberry or cherry juice concentrate

Nutrition Facts

calories	total fat	carbs	protein
276	19g	21g	9g

Notes and Suggestions

This recipe can be varied by substituting other fresh fruits in season. Even though this has no grain and is relatively low in sugars compared with most dessert recipes, you should still be watchful about how you handle the concentrated carbohydrates, especially if you're a PT. If you are just expanding your food list, you might try a very small portion (less than ⅓ of a serving) at first, then see how you do. If you find yourself craving more, then you can take this as a sign that you are still in the process of fine-tuning your food intake and that your metabolism isn't really stabilized enough to handle the more concentrated carbs. Your body will tell you.

1 preheat oven to 350°F. Grease an 8" round, layer cake pan. Grind almonds in food processor with steel blade until fine.

2 beat egg yolks until thick with wire whisk or beater in medium mixing bowl. Gradually beat in maple syrup.

3 beat egg whites in separate grease-free bowl with wire whisk or beater until foamy. Add pinch of salt and continue beating until whites are stiff, but not dry. Fold beaten egg whites into egg yolk mixture.

4 spread evenly in greased cake pan. Bake 18–20 minutes until puffy and brown. Turn off oven and leave door open, letting torte rest for about 10 minutes. After cake rests, remove from pan and place on large serving plate. Let cool.

5 spread torte with nut cream. Top with blueberries and raspberries. Drizzle with blueberry concentrate. Serve immediately.

Serves 8. Preparation time: 15 minutes.

Girls' Sprout Cookies

You'll always be prepared to create healthy treats with this handy seed mix, including these healthy goodies.

2	cups Sweet Sunny Seed Mix (page 215)
1/2	cup dried currants or dried blueberries (lower carbs than currants)
1/2	cup dry or fresh, unsweetened coconut
2	cups sunflower sprouts
3	Tbsp blueberry or cherry juice concentrate

Nutrition Facts

calories	total fat	carbs	protein
27	2g	3g	1g

1 in food processor workbowl, grind Sweet Sunny Seed Mix to crumbly texture, approx 30–45 seconds.

2 add currants or blueberries and coconut. Process for about 10–15 seconds, just to chop.

3 add sunflower sprouts and blueberry syrup and process until mixture forms a dough.

4 shape by tablespoons into balls and roll in coconut. Or shape into cookies by placing balls between layers of waxed or parchment paper and flattening with the bottom of a glass.

5 allow to dry for at least one hour. Can be eaten as is for maximum nutrition, or dehydrated for 2–3 hours at 110°F in a food dehydrator (page 73) or "baked" for 1½ hours at lowest setting of oven.

Serves 36. Preparation time: 15 minutes.

No-Flour Pie Crusts

Believe it or not, you can make savory pie crusts without flour!

1/2	cup organic flax seeds
1/2	cup organic sesame seeds
1	Tbsp organic, raw butter, cold
1/2	cup grated grass-fed Swiss or cheddar cheese
3/4	tsp ground allspice
1/2	tsp Spike vegetable seasoning or Mrs. Dash

Nutrition Facts

calories	total fat	carbs	protein
192	15g	8g	8g

Savory Crust

1 preheat oven to 375°F. In food processor workbowl. add ground flax, ground sesame seed, cold butter, shredded cheese, allspice and Spike. Pulse for 5 seconds, only until mixture starts to come together. Do not overprocess.

2 pat mixture evenly into lightly greased 8" shallow pie pan.

3 bake in preheated 375°F. oven alone for 7–10 minutes, only until crust is getting brown. If using crust for quiche or other filling, baking temperature will depend upon recipe.

Sweet Crust

1 proceed with recipe as above, except substitute 1/2 cup sesame tahini or macadamia nut butter for butter and cheese. Use 1/2 tsp nutmeg instead of Spike.

2 pat into 8" pie tin. Bake 7–10 minutes by itself, or according to recipe directions with a dessert filling. Remove from oven and let stand until cool.

Serves 6. Preparation time: 15 minutes.

No-Grain Crêpes

Crêpes are thin, flat unleavened pancakes the French have rolled around vegetables, meats, eggs, and desserts for centuries.

2	large whole eggs
1	cup whole organic milk
1/2	cup water
1/4	tsp sea salt
1/2	tsp vanilla extract
1/2	tsp grated nutmeg
1	cup Beans 'R' Us Bean Flour (page 252)
2	Tbsp melted organic butter or coconut oil

1 pour eggs, milk, water, salt, nutmeg, vanilla, flour and butter or oil into blender container. Process until just mixed, scraping down sides, if necessary. Process on medium for about 10 seconds to blend.

2 important step: Let rest for at least 30 minutes and preferably 1 hour.

3 heat a crêpe pan or heavy flat skillet over medium high until hot. Grease with a dab of oil, then pour 1/4 cup batter over hot pan, rotating pan to distribute a light coating of batter evenly. Cook crêpe until golden on the bottom and starting to dry on top, about 1–2 minutes.

4 flip crêpe with metal spatula and cook less than 1 minute more. Remove to plate to cool. Repeat procedure until all crêpe batter has been used.

5 use immediately as wrapper for meat and/or vegetable or cheese fillings, desserts, etc. or wrap tightly and refrigerate or freeze for future use.

Serves 16. Serving Size: 16–6 inch crepes. Preparation time: 10 minutes.

Nutrition Facts

calories	total fat	carbs	protein
72	6g	4g	3g

Notes and Suggestions

These delicious and handy wraps can be made successfully with alternative low-carb flour. Made ahead in a batch session, they can be stored, tightly wrapped in the freezer to be pulled out as needed for weeknight or weekend meals.

Nut Gems / Cake

Crunchy and golden on the outside, kind of soft and gooey on the inside, these are downright good, especially for being low carb and no-grain.

1⅓	cup almonds
1⅓	cup dry, unsweetened coconut
½	tsp baking soda
½	tsp salt
¾	tsp nutmeg
3	Tbsp dried currants
3	Tbsp dried blueberries
1	large egg or 2 egg whites
½	cup yogurt
3	Tbsp maple syrup
½	tsp vanilla

1 preheat oven to 325°F. In food processor workbowl, add almonds while machine is running. Process until nuts become a coarse meal, only about 30 seconds, depending upon power of machine.

2 add coconut, baking soda, salt, and nutmeg and process until mixture becomes like a grainy flour. It will not be smooth like wheat or other grain flour.

3 in small bowl or large measuring cup, combine currants, blueberries, eggs, yogurt, maple syrup, and vanilla, stirring to blend. Add to dry mixture and pulse a few times until mixture forms a batter.

4 drop by rounded tablespoons onto greased cookie sheet and flatten. Or drop into greased mini-muffin tins, or spread into a greased and lined 6" baking pan.

5 bake in preheated oven for 10–18 or 20 minutes, depending upon pan. Watch carefully. These little treats can go from golden to dark brown before you know it.

Serves 16. Preparation time: 15 minutes.

Nutrition Facts

calories	total fat	carbs	protein
118	9g	8g	4g

Notes and Suggestions

These are really good warm, reminding you of warm and chewy coconut macaroons. (They basically are.) Best results are obtained by making these into flattened cookies, balls or thimble muffins. If you make a little cake, be sure to grease the pan and line with parchment-type paper. Loosen around edges after baking, then flip onto plate, peeling off paper when slightly cool.

Nutaroons

Reminiscent of macaroons with bits of fruits and seeds, these little confections are surprisingly tasty, especially since they have no flour or oil.

1⅓	cups sunflower seeds
1⅓	cups dry, unsweetened coconut
¼	cup dried blueberries, cranberries, or currants
½	tsp baking soda
½	tsp salt
¼	tsp nutmeg
1	large egg or 2 egg whites
3	Tbsp maple syrup
3	Tbsp cherry juice concentrate
½	tsp vanilla extract
½	tsp almond extract
½	cup yogurt
	Nut Cream (optional, page 231)

1 preheat oven to 325°F. In dry workbowl of food processor with machine running on medium, add sunflower seeds. Process for about 30 seconds, or until there are only a few seed pieces still intact. Add coconut and process on medium high until mixture becomes a relatively fine, grainy flour.

2 add dried blueberries and process for 30–40 more seconds, until fruits are chopped. Whir in baking soda, salt, and nutmeg to mix. Turn off machine.

3 in small bowl or large measuring cup, combine egg or egg white, maple syrup, Cherry Concentrate, vanilla and almond extracts, and yogurt. Add liquid ingredients to flour in food processor and pulse gently a few times only, until mixture starts to form a batter. This batter thickens up as it sets, so you might find it easier to let it rest for a few minutes, while the coconut rehydrates, before forming into cookies.

4 drop by tablespoons onto greased cookie sheet or mini-muffin tins or spread into a 6–8" round pan that has been greased and lined with a parchment paper-type liner. Bake for 10–15 minutes, checking periodically. Let cool slightly, then remove carefully from pan.

5 cool to room temperature. Serve. If making a cake, cut into wedges and serve, topped with a tiny dollop of Nut Cream, if desired.

Serves 16. Preparation time: 10 minutes.

Nutrition Facts

calories	total fat	carbs	protein
73	4g	8g	2g

Notes and Suggestions

Whale this batter may be prepared in a very small cake or loaf pan, lined and greased, the mixture tends to brown readily, even at a low temperature. So, you'll probably be happier in the long run, dropping these by tablespoons and flattening them into cookies with the bottom of a glass. Watch carefully, they can burn faster than you'd like.

Piña Colada Chewies

A sweet treat for a special reward that uses up leftover pineapple juice pulp.

1	cup pineapple pulp from juicing
1/2	cup raw, organic cashews or almonds, ground
1/2	cup fresh or dry, unsweetened coconut meat shreds
2	Tbsp honey

Nutrition Facts

calories	total fat	carbs	protein
51	4g	4g	1g

1 in workbowl of food processor with steel blade, combine drained pineapple pulp, nuts, coconut meat and honey.

2 process for 45–60 seconds until well blended, but not mushy.

3 shape by tablespoons into thin 2" round patties and dehydrate at 110°F. for 12 hours in dehydrator (page 73). Can also be dried on lightly greased sheet pan at lowest oven setting for 4–5 hours.

Serves 32. Preparation time: 5 minutes.

Quick Halvah

*Halvah is a Middle Eastern candy traditionally made with sesame seed but-
ter. This quick and tasty version with alternative, low-carb ingredients and
NO sugar is a real treat.*

¼   **cup raw pecans, walnuts, almonds or cashews**

¼   **cup dried cranberries or blueberries**

¼   **cup dry or fresh unsweetened coconut shreds**

¼   **cup vanilla-flavored whey powder (page 253)**

¼   **cup raw cashew or sesame butter**

2   **tsp coconut milk or raw cream**

Nutrition Facts

calories	total fat	carbs	protein
81	4g	11g	1g

1 in blender container or food processor workbowl, add raw nuts and
dried fruit, dry coconut, whey powder and cashew butter. Process
until nuts are ground. With rubber spatula, loosen mix from bottom
of container.

2 add coconut milk and process just until mixture comes together.
Scoop by tablespoons into balls, half rounds or press into small pan
and cut into diamonds or triangles. Can serve immediately or sprinkle
with coconut shreds.

Serves 16. Preparation time: 5 minutes.

Sesame Vegetable Crackers

A tasty snack cracker you can make at home from healthy ingredients—but no flour.

2	cups hulled sesame seeds
1	cup sunflower seeds
½	cup golden flax seeds
1	med shallot or 2 garlic cloves
2	med green onions
1	tsp celery seed
1	tsp Spike vegetable seasoning or kelp
2	stalks celery, cut up
½	cup chopped parsley or fresh dillweed, packed

Nutrition Facts

calories	total fat	carbs	protein
55	4g	4g	2g

1 use organically-grown seeds, if possible. Soak sesame, sunflower and flax seeds in jar or bowl of filtered water 8–12 hours, draining and rinsing several times. Drain well by inverting jar or placing seeds in strainer.

2 in blender or food processor fitted with a steel blade, blend soaked, drained seeds in batches, if necessary, until smooth. Remove to bowl.

3 process shallot, green onions, celery seed, Spike, celery in food processor until ground. Add parsley, processing until fine. Combine vegetables with ground seeds to make a dough.

4 roll or pat dough to ¼" thickness between sheets of waxed paper. Invert onto dehydrator sheet. Score or make a grid of cuts into the dough to desired cracker size.

5 place in dehydrator (page 73) at 105°F. and dry for 8–12 hours or until crisp for "live" crackers. Or bake at lowest setting of oven for 4–6 hours, or until desired crispness. Let cool. Cut or break into pieces.

Serves 48. Preparation time: 20 minutes.

Sundried Tomato Wraps

You wouldn't know that these delicious wraps are made not with flour, but from healthy raw vegetables and seeds.

2	cups ground flax seeds, golden or brown
1½	cups water
1	tsp sea salt
3	cloves garlic
1	cup chopped fresh basil
½	med onion, chopped
1	cup sundried tomatoes
3	red bell peppers, chopped
¼	tsp cayenne pepper
2	tsp oregano

1 grind flax seeds in a spice grinder or blender.

2 place all remaining ingredients, except water and ground flax seeds in a blender or food processor and blend.

3 add water and ground flax, and blend until smooth. Allow to sit for 30 minutes to thicken.

4 spread thinly into circles on teflex-lined dehydrator sheets, and dehydrate (page 73) at 105°F. for about 6 hours, or until easily removed from the teflex. Flip onto mesh sheets, and dry for an additional 4 hours, or until dry but still flexible.

5 allow to cool, then store in plastic bags in the refrigerator for up to a month.

Serves 8. Preparation time: 15 minutes.

Nutrition Facts

calories	total fat	carbs	protein
228	14g	21g	9g

Notes and Suggestions

These no-flour, dehydrated raw food wraps can be used in place of tortillas or other flat bread folded over a wide variety of vegetable, meat, cheese and other fillings. They make a hearty lunch, served with guacamole or hummus, lettuce, tomato, and sprouts. Vegetable wrap recipe, courtesy Enchanted Kitchens, Raw Foods Chef, Jenny Cornbleet.

Zucchini Muffins

You might be surprised to learn that it is possible to make good-tasting muffins without grain flour.

3	cups blanched almond flour*
2	tsp cinnamon
1	tsp nutmeg
1	tsp baking soda
½	tsp salt
3	med eggs, beaten
⅓	cup melted butter or coconut oil
¼	cup honey
2–3	drops lemon oil or ½ tsp grated lemon peel
3	cups grated zucchini

1 preheat oven to 350°F. Line muffin cups with paper liners.

2 mix almond flour, cinnamon, nutmeg, baking soda, and salt in mixing bowl.

3 add beaten eggs, butter, honey, lemon, and grated zucchini. Stir to blend.

4 divide batter into muffin tins, but do not overfill. Works better with smaller muffins.

5 bake for approximately 15 minutes, or until done. Remove from oven and let cool slightly on wire racks.

Serves 24. Preparation time: 15 minutes.

Nutrition Facts

calories	total fat	carbs	protein
154	13g	8g	5g

Cooking Tips

*Almond flour can made be easily at home with a food processor or juicer or purchased ready made from specialty vendors you can find starting on page 249. In small quantities, making almond flour from the nuts with their skins on is okay for everyday consumption, but when using larger quantities in baked goods and desserts, it's better to skin them to avoid large quantities of tannins and enzyme inhibitors.

To de-skin almonds: Pour boiling water over almonds in a jar or bowl. Let stand until water cools to tolerable temperature, then slip off almond skins by holding between thumb and index finger and squeezing. Skins should slip off easily, but watch out for flying projectiles! Dry by patting gently with paper towel.

To make almond flour: Grind dry, skinned almonds in food processor by starting with a dry workbowl, then adding almonds into running machine through feed tube. Process until almonds are finely ground into a meal or flour. It will not be as smooth or fine as white flour. Store in covered container in refrigerator or freezer. Keeps up to 3 months in freezer.

Notes and Suggestions

This is a high calorie recipe that would probably satisfy a fast oxidizing PT type, but would not be conducive for someone trying to lose weight.

THE RECIPES: Snacks & Handhelds

Snack time is usually a fun eating time. That is, unless you are caught empty-handed while away from home without the foods you need. Snacks are an important part of the Total Health Program. They help keep blood sugar levels stable and are helpful for fine-tuning your diet. They should be planned into your food schedule with as much attention as full meals. Remember, you are retraining your body and how it relates to food. Carbohydrate Types find they can often go for long periods of time without eating. But they need to be just as diligent about planning and eating snacks as Protein Types, who need to eat more frequently because of their fast metabolism.

Snack Recipes and Ideas

You will find many food recipes and ideas for snacking in this "Snacks and Handhelds" section, and in "Raw, Sprouted and Fermented Foods," "Juices and Shakes," and "Condiments and Extras," but actually any of the recipes in this book could be served as snacks, so think "leftovers!" Actually, it's a good strategy to be more proactive and plan what snacks you will be taking. This way you will always be prepared, will feel confident and won't psychologically or literally ever be "out of luck" without the best foods for yourself within easy reach. Of course, it's not about luck. It's all about paying attention and planning.

Snack Pack

An excellent strategy is to assemble and maintain a "Snack Kit" to carry with you, containing a store of the ideal foods for your specific metabolic type. These might include small single serving containers of nut butters, trail or fuel mixes, vegetable and fruit leathers, cubes of cheese, meat, sprouts, and/or leftovers from meals. Here is a list of snack ideas. Some of these are recipes in this section, others are recipes elsewhere in this cookbook, and some (those where not all words are capitalized) are simple snacks you can create in seconds, like celery & cheese. These snack ideas are presented from those most ideal for Protein Types to those most ideal for Carb Types.

    Stuffed mushrooms
    Celery & nut butter
    Celery & cheese
    Celery & dark turkey
    Jicama & bison summer sausage
    Crunchy Sprout Mixes
    Roll-Ups
    Marinated Italian Salad
    Basic or Savory Sunny Seeds
    Avocado and Sesame Spread

Roast beef & sprouts
Salmon Seviche
Fresh Coconut Chunks
Walnut Paté
PT's Cruiser
Hardcooked Eggs
Kohlrabi and Side Kickers Veggies with Seed Dip
Pickles and Jicama
Rainbow Coleslaw w/Seeds Mexican Live 'n Kickin' Bean Dip with sprouts
Cheese bread with fresh herbs
Hummus spread with red peppers
Middle Eastern Salad
Egg Foo Yung with lettuce, tomato, mayo
Egg Salad with Artichokes
Sweet Sunny Seed Mix
Grilled Ratatouille
Raw Vegetables
Cup o' Vegetable Soup
Sprout Pate
Crunchy Herb Sprout Mix
Gazpacho Soup
Roll-Ups with lettuce, sprouts
Cut up Vegetable Sticks
Vegetable Leathers
Vegetable Crispers
Eggplant Cheeseburgers
Stuffed Eggs
Sea Salad Side
Stuffed Cukes and Zukes
Sesame Vegetable Crackers
Sprouts, Sprouts, Sprouts

Roll-Ups

"Life without bread? What am I going to eat instead of a sandwich for lunch?" This is probably one of the biggest challenges to embracing and incorporating a no-grain, low-carb lifestyle. The Fourth Earl of Sandwich undoubtedly hit upon a popular totable when he stuffed meat between two slabs of bread, but there are lots more varied, interesting—and healthy—things to eat for your meals and snacks. And your body will love it.

The term sandwich is actually a verb, as well as a noun. "To sandwich" also means to "insert or squeeze between two other things," and the definition includes "something that resembles a sandwich." Even though typical, there is no requirement that a sandwich has to be made from wheat or rye. Instead try these:

Types of Wrappers
Butter lettuce leaves
Boston lettuce leaves
Red and Green leaf lettuces
Romaine lettuce
Cabbage leaves
Collard leaves
Kale leaves
Wide, thin Zucchini Strips
Wide, thin Cucumber Strips
Steamed Eggplant slices
Celery stalks
Stuffed Cukes and Zukes
Pickled Grape leaves
No-Grain Flat breads
No-Grain Dehydrated Wraps
No-Grain Crêpes
No-Grain Waffles
No-Grain Pie Crusts
Thin Omelets
Egg Foo Yung
Nori Seaweed Sheets
Slices of Meat
Slices of Cheese
Parmesan Crisps
Vegetable Leathers

Styles of Wraps: Wrap and Roll

Rolled: Lay wrapper flat, fill or spread with about 2–3 Tbsp filling, then fold wrapper over filling, rolling up tightly jellyroll style.

Burrito style: Lay wrapper flat, spread or fill with desired filling; fold opposites sides inward one-fourth to one-third of the way on each side, fold wrapper over filling, rolling up tightly into "bundle." Place edge side down on plate or pan.

Cones: Roll Nori or square wrapper into a cone, with one wide-open end. Moisten narrow end edge with water to seal. Spoon or place base filling into cone, then press around and up the sides to cover inside, making room for additional vegetables, meats, sprouts etc.

Flat, Tostada-Style: For crisper or less flexible wraps, simply lay wrap or crisp on plate, spread with topping, additional vegetables or sprouts, condiments and or garnish and serve.

Fillings (An endless array...)
> Vegetables, cut up, grated
> Nut Butters & Creams
> Fillings & Spreads
> Sprouts or Sprout mixes
> Sliced Meats, Tempeh, Sliced or Blended Cheeses
> Leftover Casseroles
> Salads and Slaws
> Leftover Stir-Fry

Basic Sunny Seed Mix Plus

This versatile, complete protein seed mix can be the starting point for an almost endless array of sweet and savory low-carb snacks, shakes, trail mixes and toppers.

1⅓ **cup sunflower seeds, organic**

⅓ **cup sesame seeds, organic**

⅓ **cup pumpkin seeds, (green pepitas)**

⅓ **cup flax seeds, organic**

1 combine seeds.

2 store covered in refrigerator or freezer for up to two months.

Serves 32. Serving Size: 1 Tbsp per serving. Preparation time: 5 minutes.

Nutrition Facts

calories	total fat	carbs	protein
35	3g	2g	1g

sunny seed mix variations

Sweet Sunny Seed Mix

to Basic Sunny Seed Mix, add ⅔ cup dry, unsweetened coconut, ¼ cup finely chopped dried currants, 1 tsp nutmeg and ½ tsp ground cinnamon. Store in tightly covered glass jar in refrigerator or freezer.

Savory Sunny Seed Mix

in heavy dry, cast iron skillet over medium heat, lightly toast Basic Sunny Seed Mix, stirring constantly, until pumpkin seeds start to pop and aroma of lightly toasted sesame appears. Remove from heat.

add ⅓ cup dry mixed vegetables (soup mix) that have been whirred to powdery in blender, 1½ Tbsp poultry seasoning, 1½ Tbsp debittered nutritional yeast, and 1 tsp Spike vegetable seasoning or Mrs Dash. Stir, cool, and store in container with lid in refrigerator for up to six weeks.

Sunny Seed Gomasio

blend 1 recipe Savory Sunny Seed Mix, above, in blender until it becomes a fine powder. Store in covered container in refrigerator. Use as a topping or seasoning.

Sprouted Sunny Seed Mix

place Basic Sunny Seed Mix in glass jar. Cover with water. Cover with mesh screen or cheesecloth and secure with rubber band or screw lid. Soak 5–8 hours or overnight. Drain and rinse. Let seeds "sprout" for 3 hours. Rinse and drain again. Use as salad, snack, or base for Roll-Up or sandwich filling.

Chewy Nutsy "Cereal"

When you're hankering for a bowl of cereal or chewy grains, try this taste and texture match for a quick breakfast or snack.

¼   cup whole organic flax seeds
¼   cup raw organic almonds or walnuts
¼   cup dry, unsweetened coconut
2   tsp dried mint leaves or 2 mint tea bags
1   cup coconut milk

Nutrition Facts

calories	total fat	carbs	protein
315	28g	14g	6g

Notes and Suggestions

Made up ahead and kept on hand in the refrigerator, it can also be used as base for low-carb, no-grain "gorp" balls and other treats. This is a high-calorie, high-fat recipe, not appropriate for weight loss.

1 in dry blender or food processor with motor running, pour flax seeds, almonds, and dry coconut through opening in top of cover. Replace removable cap and continue processing until ingredients are reduced to a chunky, grain-like consistency, about 1 minute.

2 stop motor, scrape down to loosen mixture in bottom of blender or workbowl, if necessary. Add loose, dry mint leaves or open 2 mint tea bags and dump contents. Process a few bursts more until blended.

3 scoop out ¼ cup mixture per serving. Pour roughly equal amount, ¼–⅓ cup coconut milk or other nut milk per serving over "cereal" and enjoy.

4 can be enjoyed cold, or let stand a few minutes and warm slightly on stovetop for a "hot" cereal experience. Flax seeds will thicken mixture as it sits. Nutrition at peak served cold.

Serves 4. Serving size: ¼ cup minimum serving plus milk.
Preparation time: 5 minutes.

Nori Bruschetta

A hybrid of Italian and Japanese tastes, this unique, colorful, appetizer snack is as stunning as it is healthy and delicious.

4	sheets nori seaweed
2	med tomatoes, chopped
1	med garlic clove, minced
2	med scallions or green onions, chopped
1/2	cup mung bean or clover-radish sprouts, chopped
1/2	cup chopped Italian flat-leaf parsley
1	Tbsp extra virgin olive oil
1/2	tsp Spike vegetable seasoning or Bragg's
2–3	grinds freshly ground black pepper

Nutrition Facts

calories	total fat	carbs	protein
12	1g	1g	0g

Notes and Suggestions

A great snack or appetizer for a CT, or anyone for that matter. PT's will, of course, want to enjoy this with some additional protein to make it a balanced snack.

1 toast nori sheets by passing over burner, preferably gas, on high. Nori will turn greenish black and stiffen. Cut nori sheets with scissors into 2 to 2½" squares.

2 make bruschetta by combining chopped tomatoes, garlic, scallions, mung bean sprouts, and parsley with olive oil, Spike, and pepper in large mixing bowl. Drain off liquid.

3 place stacks of two toasted nori squares together on serving platter.

4 make sure bruschetta mixture is drained well. Mound approximately 1½ Tbsp bruschetta mixture on top of each nori square stack. If desired, sprinkle with a little Parmesan cheese or sesame seeds. Serve immediately.

Serves 18. Serving Size: 1 square. Preparation time: 15 minutes.

Parmesan Crisps

These simple, yet innovative crisps can substitute for taco shells, crackers and flatbreads in a variety of applications.

1   **cup shredded (not grated) Parmesan cheese**

1   **tsp paprika**

Nutrition Facts

calories	total fat	carbs	protein
54	4g	1g	5g

Notes and Suggestions

If planning to use this for larger purposes like taco shell substitute, make crisps larger with 2 or more Tbsp cheese. Note: Grated Parmesan cheese will NOT work in this recipe. For the results you want, you need to use high-quality shredded Parmesan or Parmesan-Romano blend.

1 preheat oven to 375°F. On cookie sheet lined with parchment paper or silpat liner (reusable silicon), spread about 1 Tbsp shredded Parmesan cheese evenly into circles about 4–5" each. Sprinkle with paprika.

2 bake in preheated 375°F. oven for 5–8 minutes, until golden brown. Cheese will melt together and form disks. Remove from oven and let rest until crisps have cooled.

3 using a flat spatula, carefully lift crisps to serving platter or into covered container. Crisps can also be formed around a bottle right out of the oven to create taco-like shells.

Serves 16. Preparation time: 10 minutes.

PT's Cruiser

This quick, hearty salad could be a real pick-me-up for a PT's afternoon snack.

1	cup finely chopped celery
1	cup diced fresh or canned asparagus
1	cup artichokes, diced
1	can sardines, drained and chopped
4	anchovy filets, packed in olive oil
1	Tbsp chopped capers or finely chopped dill pickle
2	tsp olive oil from anchovies
1	tsp fresh lemon juice

1 in small mixing bowl or storage container, combine finely chopped celery, asparagus, artichoke hearts, sardines, anchovies, capers, olive oil, and lemon juice. Stir to combine ingredients evenly.

2 this could also be prepared fast in a food processor, if you are careful not to overmix. Start by adding celery and processing until finely chopped. Turn off machine, then add asparagus and artichoke hearts, pulse with a few on and off bursts to chop. Stop machine. Add sardines and anchovies, capers, olive oil, and lemon juice. Pulse one or two more times. DO NOT overmix.

3 makes 2 servings. Or serve half for a snack today and half for next day's lunch. Store what's left in covered container. Refrigerate for up to 1 day.

Serves 2. Preparation time: 10 minutes.

Nutrition Facts

calories	total fat	carbs	protein
277	14g	14g	26g

Cooking Tips

PT or MX: The name says PT, but MX could also enjoy this, perhaps for a lunch salad.

Notes and Suggestions

This fish and vegetable salad could easily be a mini-meal or the protein complement for a lunch meal for PT or MX. Add a Basic Vegetable Soup or Cream of Mushroom Soup for a whole meal.

Quick Yogurt Cup

A quick, simple snack.

½	cup plain organic yogurt
1	Tbsp raw or organic half and half
1	Tbsp ready-to-drink Chai tea

Nutrition Facts

calories	total fat	carbs	protein
99	6g	8g	5g

1 spoon yogurt into serving cup or dish.

2 pour over cream and Chai tea. Enjoy.

Serves 1. Preparation time: 1 minute.

Cooking Tips

PT: Definitely more of a PT type snack, especially with the cream. You may want some nuts to make this a balanced snack for you.

CT: Since your metabolic type should limit dairy and fat, plan to consume this only once in a while without the cream, using lowfat yogurt.

Notes and Suggestions

Try substituting 1 tsp Cherry or Blueberry Concentrate (page 253) for the Chai tea. Monitor carefully whether even these high quality fruit juice concentrates elevate your blood sugar too much, making you tired or hungry later. Try eating this snack with more protein, possibly sprinkling with 1–2 tsp nuts or Sunny Seed Mix.

Sesame Miso Spread

This deceptively simple spread is a versatile base for making snacks, spreads, fillings, salad dressings, and sauces.

1	cup raw tahini or mechanically-hulled sesame butter
1½	Tbsp light miso, fermented soybean paste
1	clove garlic, minced
1	Tbsp hot water
2	Tbsp chopped scallion

1 measure raw tahini into small measuring bowl or container with cover. Stir in miso and minced garlic to blend.

2 stir in hot water a little at a time, and stir until mixture becomes smooth. Mixture will seize up initially, then become smooth and glossy.

3 stir in chopped scallions. Cover and store in refrigerator.

Serves 16. Serving size: about 1 Tbsp. Preparation time: 5 minutes.

Nutrition Facts

calories	total fat	carbs	protein
90	8g	3g	3g

Cooking Tips

While this is a good PT type snack because of the protein and fat, CT's can also enjoy it from time to time with added vegetables as mentioned below.

Notes and Suggestions

Keep this basic spread in your refrigerator or tote it along with celery and zucchini sticks for a handy snack. It can also become the base for sandwich fillings by adding grated vegetables such as zucchini, carrot, sprouts.

Snazzy Gingered Nuts

Savory and spicy, these roasted nuts are a special treat, good enough for company, if there's any left....

¼	cup raw organic butter
⅓	cup tamari soy sauce
2	tsp ground ginger powder
¼	tsp Japanese hot wasabi paste, if desired
2	cups organic walnuts
1	cup organic almonds or pecans
1	cup raw macadamia nuts or cashews

Nutrition Facts

calories	total fat	carbs	protein
59	6g	1g	1g

Cooking Tips

While PT's can enjoy nuts as a snack or protein food, CT's will want to limit their use, since they are proportionately too high in fat for your metabolic type or anyone focused on weight loss. Note the 1 Tbsp serving size.

1 preheat oven to 300°F. Melt butter in small saucepan over low. Combine soy sauce, ginger and wasabi paste (fiery, green sushi condiment) in small bowl.

2 spread nuts over cookie sheet or 9"x13" baking pan. Pour on butter and stir to coat. Bake for about 15 minutes.

3 remove from oven. Stir in ginger-soy mixture. Return to oven and roast about 10 minutes more. Remove from oven. Stop. You have to let these cool BEFORE you eat them.

4 let stand at room temperature to cool. Store in a covered container. Use within a few days, as if that will be a problem...

Serves 64. Serving Size: 1 Tbsp per serving. Preparation time: 10 minutes.

Vegetable Crispers

These baked or dehydrated vegetable "chips" may not be as fancy as those commercial potato or perfectly-shaped grain chips, but they'll give you snacking satisfaction on a low-carb budget.

1	med eggplant, cut into ⅛–¼" slices
2	med zucchinis, cut diagonally into ⅛–¼" slices
2	med kohlrabi, peeled, halved and cut into ⅛–¼" slices
1	med jicama, peeled and cut into ⅛–¼" slices
1	cup green beans, snapped and halved
1	Tbsp grapeseed or olive oil
2	tsp tamari soy sauce

1 cut eggplant first. Some larger eggplants may be bitter, so tossing slices with 1 tsp salt, then letting them set while preparing other vegetables, will draw out bitter liquid. Rinse off briny liquid and pat slices dry.

2 place equal sized, dry vegetable slices in large mixing bowl. Pour oil and tamari over vegetable slices, tossing to coat evenly.

3 place coated slices on dehydrator screens (page 73) or on lightly greased cookie sheet. Dehydrate at 110°F. for 4–8 hours or at lowest setting of oven for 3–4 hours, until vegetables are dried and crunchy, leathery or chewy-crunchy. Zucchini or thicker slices may require 7–10 hours in dehydrator.

4 cool. Remove to tight-fitting covered jar. Store at room temperature for 3–4 weeks.

Serves 8. Preparation time: 20 minutes.

Nutrition Facts

calories	total fat	carbs	protein
85	2g	16g	3g

Cooking Tips

PT: Emphasize the lower starch vegetables recommended for your type (like green beans, cauliflower, celery), then experiment with trying other veggies, as your body gets more aligned with your own naturally healthy state.

CT: You have a wider variety of allowable vegetables to start with, but essentially the same process hold true for you.

Notes and Suggestions

A variety of vegetables can be used to make these "snackers", which can be served as snack chips or crackers with dips or spreads, or to accompany soup or salad. See page 254 for dehydrator manufacturers. These, by no stretch of the imagination, are like commercial crackers and/or snack chips. But they are flavorful and nutritious and can fill a need for occasional snacking. But if you're "craving" junk food, take it as a sign that you'd best try some EFT first.

Vegetable Leathers

Like fruit leathers, vegetable leathers made by dehydrating blended, leftover vegetables or even gazpacho soup can be a nutritious, on-the-go snack.

4   cups lightly steamed, puréed (blended) vegetables OR
       gazpacho or other blended, non-dairy fresh vegetable soup

Nutrition Facts

calories	total fat	carbs	protein
25	0g	4.5g	0g

Notes and Suggestions

See page 254 for suppliers of dehydrators and other recommended kitchen equipment.

To dehydrate vegetable leathers in food dehydrator:

1 pour about 4 cups fresh vegetable purée onto plastic wrapped screens or Teflon/Teflex lined trays. Dehydrate at 135°F. for 5–6 hours until somewhat glossy and no longer sticky. Remove. Cool. Snip into quarters. Roll up and wrap tightly. Store in dry place.

To dehydrate vegetable leathers in oven:

1 grease cookie sheet very lightly with coconut oil. Spread 3–4 cups thick vegetable purée or soup evenly over surface, a little thicker at edges.

2 turn oven to lowest possible setting and dehydrate vegetables until dry, as described above. When firm, remove, cool and snip into desired pieces. Roll up and tightly wrap. Store in a dry place.

Serves 8. Serving size: 1 Roll-Up. Preparation time: 15 minutes.

THE RECIPES: Raw, Sprouted & Fermented Foods

This chapter honors and embraces the oldest and healthiest of all types of foodstuffs. Long before modern refrigeration, people throughout history have not only existed, but thrived, on the culturing or fermenting of dairy products, vegetables, seeds and other foods.

Live, sprouted and fermented foods all have superior nutritional benefits. Heat used in cooking and commercial food processing methods "sterilizes" food, making it "shelf stable," but can destroy and deactivate important nutrients like many vitamins and enzymes that are especially critical in the digestion and utilization of the foods we eat. Eating more high quality, organic, raw, sprouted and fermented foods, on the other hand, actually ensures more B vitamins, enzymes and better digestion. You'll be surprised at how simple and easy these recipes are to produce.

Sprouting Guidelines

Sprouting is a simple, low-cost way to obtain high-quality, live food, regardless of the season. It is an easy process that can literally explode the life-supporting nutrition of the original seed, which contains all the genetic material and initial food the plant needs to start its life. Obviously sprouting is a highly beneficial practice. It is the cornerstone of a raw food diet, and one you need to learn so you can regularly enhance your own.

The Chinese discovered the value of sprouting seeds, which they used as life-giving food, and to avoid scurvy on long ocean voyages. Germinating seeds not only yields the vitamin C that prevents this disease, but neutralizes anti-factors such as phytic acid and enzyme inhibitors that interrupt the absorption of nutrients. Starchy carbs are reduced, nutrients become predigested and, along with enzymes, are dramatically increased from seed to sprout.

Some of the most popular sprouts are alfalfa, almond, broccoli, clover, flax, garbanzo, lentil, mung bean, pumpkin, onion, radish, sesame and sunflower. Actually any raw seed, nut or bean can be sprouted alone or mixed with others. Alfalfa is the most popular commercial sprout, and probably the one with which you are most familiar. But don't restrict yourself or your tastes. Many sprouts have much more interesting flavor and higher nutrition than alfalfa. In fact, some nutritional authorities recommend avoidance of alfalfa sprouts due to the presence of toxins.

Method for Growing Sprouts

Seeds differ in length of time needed to sprout, but the basic method for sprouting them is generally the same. Rinsing is the key for successful sprouts.

1. Place seeds in glass jar and cover with clean, fresh, filtered water, preferably with cheesecloth or mesh screen secured over opening. In a quart mason jar, add $1\frac{1}{2}$ Tbsp seeds or $\frac{1}{4}$ cup beans or $\frac{1}{2}$ cup nuts, and about four times that volume of water. In a gallon jar, add $1\frac{1}{2}$ cup seeds or 1 cup beans, legumes or nuts, with twice their volume of water.

2. Soak 5–8 hours or overnight.

3. Drain off water and rinse. Drain again.

4. Rinsing is the key. Twice a day, morning and evening, rinse and drain.

5. Keep in a dark place for 24 hours, rinsing twice a day.

6. For long sprout tails and nutritious green tips, place the jars in the light for 2–5 days, depending upon seed. Most are best after 2–3 days. Sprout times for the various seeds are as follows: clover, radish, broccoli, onion seeds: 3–4 days; beans: 3–4 days; legumes like lentils: 2–3 days; nuts and crunchy bean mixes: 3 hours. Seeds such as sunflowers with large hulls should be immersed in water so the hulls can be removed as they float to the top, or eat one at a time and manually remove hulls. If you buy commercial sprouts, rinse immediately and eat within a day.

Menu Ideas for Sprouts

Sprouts can be used in salads, spreads, soups, stews, vegetable dishes and main dishes, even shakes and juicing. Begin by sprouting and experimenting with the ones that appeal to you most. Broccoli and radish seeds are spicier, so use smaller amounts. Short sprouts like nuts and crunchy beans without tails are excellent for snack mixes. For maximum digestibility, soak your nuts and seeds for shakes, milks and spreads.

Basic Sauerkraut Plus

Sauerkraut, which translates from German as "Salt Cabbage," is a healthy, fermented food that can be served as vegetable or condiment.

2	**lbs shredded green cabbage (about 2 quarts, loosely packed)**
2	**Tbsp sea salt**
1	**tsp caraway or cumin seeds**
2	**cups clean, filtered water**

1 wash and drain cabbage. Be sure to slice thinly with a sharp knife, including core. Place in large bowl and mash or pound with a heavy cup, pestle or mallet until cabbage starts to release juice.

2 sprinkle with seeds and mix. Pack tightly into 2 quart mason jars. Stir salt into water and pour over cabbage, adding more water to bring level up within 3/4" from top of jar. Cover with lid. Store at room temperature for at least 3 days, then place in refrigerator.

Serves 32. Serving size: 2 quarts, 1/4 cup per serving.
Preparation time: 15 minutes.

sauerkraut variations

Veggie Sauerkraut

follow directions above, except use 4 cups shredded cabbage, 2 cups peeled, shredded carrot, 1 cup french style green beans, and 1 cup peeled and shredded turnips.

South American Sauerkraut

follow directions above, adding 2 medium crescent-sliced onions (cut in half lengthwise, then sliced thinly) and 3/4 tsp chili or red pepper flakes to cabbage.

Japanese Sauerkraut

follow directions above, except add 2 cloves sliced garlic, 2 Tbsp peeled and grated ginger root and 2 Tbsp tamari soy sauce.

Nutrition Facts

calories	total fat	carbs	protein
7	0g	2g	0g

Notes and Suggestions

This pickled vegetable and its variations can be made and stored for months in refrigerator or cold cellar. Use for flavor and nutrition as a vegetable side dish, condiment, addition to stews and casseroles such as Beef Pot Roast with Sauerkraut. The fermentation process makes the vegetables more digestible for all types. Recipe adapted from Sally Fallon's Nourishing Traditions, one of the most authoritative sources of information on the benefits of traditionally fermented foods.

Crème Fraîche

The French use this expensive, ultra silky "clotted cream" like sour cream in recipes, but it's easy and much healthier to make your own at home.

1 **pint high-quality raw cream, NOT ultrapasteurized**

2 **Tbsp cultured buttermilk**

1 use local, raw or organic unpasteurized cream. Place into clean glass or ceramic container, not metal or plastic.

2 add buttermilk, cover and place container in a warm, room temperature place for about 24 hours. Chill.

Serves 32. Serving size: 1 Tbsp per serving. Preparation time: 5 minutes.

Nutrition Facts

calories	total fat	carbs	protein
52	6g	0.5g	0.5g

Notes and Suggestions

This healthier dairy product can be used interchangeably with sour cream, whipped cream or mascarpone in recipes. Recipe adapted from Sally Fallon and Mary Enig's Nourishing Traditions, a highly recommended source for more information on traditional foods.

Crunchy Herb Sprout Snack Mix

This seasoned sprout mix is a healthy, crunchy, take-along snack, salad, or Roll-Up filling ingredient.

Sprout Snack Mix

2	cups mung bean sprouts
1	cup lentil sprouts
1	cup sunflower seed sprouts
½	cup garbanzo sprouts
½	cup clover sprouts
½	cup radish sprouts
½	cup grated carrot

Herb Seasoning

2	tsp thyme leaves
2	tsp oregano
1	tsp marjoram leaves
½	tsp ground rosemary
1	tsp garlic powder
1	tsp Spike vegetable seasoning or Mrs. Dash
1	tsp extra virgin olive oil

1 mix sprouts together in large bowl.

2 mix herbs and seasonings, except olive oil, together in small jar. Sprinkle 1 Tbsp of herb seasoning over sprouts in bowl. Store any remaining herb seasoning in capped jar for another time or other uses.

3 drizzle sprout mixture with olive oil and toss to mix. Serve immediately.

Serves 6. Serving Size: 1 cup per serving. Preparation time: 10 minutes.

Nutrition Facts

calories	total fat	carbs	protein
147	6g	19g	8g

Cooking Tips

This crunchy live snack mix is healthy and brimming with nutrients, good for all types. Sprout your own seeds, if possible, using organically-grown seeds, whenever possible.

PT: May still want to consume this with some meat protein, even as a snack, but try this out for yourself and see. Try with slices of buffalo summer sausage or Roll-Up as a filling in thinly sliced, grass-fed roast beef.

CT: Will probably find that the protein value is high enough to sustain you for a snack or part of a main meal.

Notes and Suggestions

Use as a finger food snack, a salad ingredient on lettuce-lined salad plate or as a Roll-Up filling, rolled into butter lettuce or cabbage leaf. Recipe suggestion courtesy The Sproutpeople. See page 252 for ordering organic seeds and sprouting equipment from this reliable source.

Mexican Live 'n Kickin' Bean Dip

Sprouted version of the popular Mexican bean dip tastes good, but struts a bonus—it's alive and kickin'!

2	cups mung bean sprouts
2	med avocados, peeled and seeded
1	med cucumber, peeled and seeded
1	Tbsp dark miso, soybean paste
1	med garlic clove
1½	Tbsp ground cumin seed
1	tsp chili powder
1	jalapeño pepper, seeded and chopped

Nutrition Facts

	calories	total fat	carbs	protein
Mixed Type:	67	5g	5g	2g
Carb Type:	40	3g	4g	1g
Protein Type:	81	6g	6g	2g

Cooking Tips

PT: Experiment to see how you feel eating this dip, with higher than normal protein for a snack, but increase portion size by serving 10 with this recipe. You may still need to eat some meat protein to feel satisfied.

CT: Try eating this as a snack, reducing avocado to 1. You may find that it suits you fine.

Notes and Suggestions

Sprouting beans reduces the carbs and increases the nutrition. Serve this healthier version of everyone's favorite bean dip as a snack or part of a meal platter with raw vegetable sticks, Vegetable Crispers or Vegetable Leathers.

1 in blender or food processor, blend bean sprouts with avocado, cucumber, miso, garlic, cumin, chili powder, and jalapeño until smooth. Add salt to taste, if desired.

2 serve as dip or pile with other ingredients into low-carb wrap, cabbage or lettuce Roll-Up.

3 can use 1½ to 2 Tbsp Mexican or taco seasoning to replace cumin, garlic, chili powder and jalapeño.

Serves 12. Serving Size: about ¼ cup per serving. Preparation time: 10 minutes.

Nut Cream

Use this creamy concoction as pudding, sauce or "whipped" topping on fruit or other "sweet" treats.

1	cup raw cashews or deskinned raw almonds, organic, if possible
½	cup cold, filtered water
1	tsp honey or ¼ packet SteviaPlus alternative sweetener (page 253)

1 blend cashews, cold water, and sweetener in blender container on high until smooth and creamy.

2 chill. Serve small 2–3 Tbsp portion as pudding or 1 Tbsp as a topping like whipped cream for fruit or dessert. Store in tightly covered container. Refrigerate. Use within two days.

Serves 16. Serving size: generally 1 Tbsp per serving. Preparation time: 5 minutes.

Nutrition Facts

calories	total fat	carbs	protein
82	7g	4g	3g

Cooking Tips

PT: This is a good for you as a snack or topping, since the higher fat and protein agrees with your metabolic type's needs.

CT: Very rich for you, as nuts are only an occasional or rare treat for your type, to be consumed sparingly and in small quantities.

Seed Cheese

A creamy, non-dairy "cheese" spread can be made simply from a combination of soaked and sprouted seeds.

2	cups raw organic sunflower seeds
1/4	cup unhulled, raw organic sesame seeds
1	cup raw organic almonds

Nutrition Facts

calories	total fat	carbs	protein
140	14g	4g	5g

Notes and Suggestions

While creamy and rich, this sprouted seed "cream" cheese can be used as a substitute from time to time as a non-dairy base for fillings, wraps, salad dressings, dips, and confections. The sprouting process makes the seeds more digestible. Feel free to add Spike, Bragg's, herbs or nutritional yeast for flavor.

1 rinse seeds, then place sunflowers and sesame seeds in large glass jar. Place almonds in separate smaller glass jar. Cover with clean, filtered water. Let soak overnight.

2 rinse and let seeds sprout for 3 hours only. Pour hot water over almonds, let soak for a few minutes, then slip off skins by holding between thumb and index finger.

3 grind drained, soaked seeds and nuts together in food processor or put through juicer until smooth.

4 place in covered container and refrigerate. Stores up to 3 days.

Serves 32. Serving Size: 2 Tbsp per serving. Preparation time: 10 minutes.

Sunny Sprout Paté

Another use for the versatile Basic Sunny Seed Mix, this time in a savory, live paté for spreads, dips or Roll-Up fillings.

2	cups Basic Sunny Seed Mix (page 215)
1/2	med red onion, coarsely chopped
1	stalk celery, stringed, cut up
2	Tbsp tamari soy sauce or Bragg's Liquid Amino's
1/2	cup coarsely chopped lemon or basil or fresh oregano, or flat-leaf parsley
1/2	tsp Spike vegetable seasoning or Mrs. Dash
3–4	grinds freshly ground black pepper

1 soak Sunny Seed Mix in covered bowl of clean, filtered water. Allow to soak at room temperature for 6–12 hours. Drain, rinse thoroughly, and rinse again.

2 add soaked, drained seeds and red onion, celery, tamari, herbs, Spike, and pepper to food processor workbowl, fitted with a metal blade. Process until smooth.

3 edible right away, but much better if refrigerated for at least 1 hour before serving. Keeps up to 3 days, covered in refrigerator.

Serves 16. Preparation time: 10 minutes.

Nutrition Facts

	calories	total fat	carbs	protein
Mixed Type:	90	7g	6g	2g
Carb Type:	45	3g	6g	2g
Protein Type:	90	7g	6g	2g

Cooking Tips

PT: This is an ideal snack for you. Increase celery to 2–3 stalks.

CT: The sprouted seeds are more digestible, but still high in fat for your type. Use only half of the sprouted seeds, add 1 coarsely grated carrot and 3/4 cup chopped parsley.

Notes and Suggestions

Serving suggestion: Spread on cabbage or lettuce leaves, top with chopped tomato and roll up as a sandwich alternative. Or serve as a dip with raw vegetable crudité.

Zucchetti Pasta

This amazing angel hair "pasta" is made from raw zucchini or yellow squash with a special Spiral Slicer you can find on page 253.

2	med zucchini or yellow squash
1/2	tsp extra virgin olive oil or raw or organic butter
1/2	tsp Spike or Mrs. Dash vegetable seasoning

Nutrition Facts

calories	*total fat*	*carbs*	*protein*
42	2g	7g	2g

Cooking Tips

Add protein to make this a balanced meal.

Notes and Suggestions

Angel hair pasta made from zucchini or other vegetables is possible using a special Spiral Slicer, a manual slicer that can make long thin strands and various other decorative and functional cuts. See page 253 for ordering this through the mail. You'll be happy you made the investment in this little gadget. You can use this ingenious device to produce an excellent vegetable noodle or spaghetti substitute for a wide variety of dishes such as spaghetti or tomato sauce, Sukiyaki with Beef or salads or other dishes calling for pasta. Excellent topped with freshly made, raw tomato sauce in the summer.

1 wash zucchini, cut into 3–4 inch cuts and secure in Spiral Slicer set to make strands. Then carefully turn handle to create one or many long continuous strands.

2 this can be eaten raw, as is, or just barely warmed (not cooked) in a little extra virgin olive oil or melted butter and Spike in a saucepan. One zucchini makes about 1 serving or 2 cups angel hair zucchetti.

3 while this device produces amazingly authentic looking pasta out of vegetables and can be used for decorative and other slicing, you can also create a pasta-like noodle by using a vegetable parer and making long thin strips of zucchini or other vegetable.

Serves 2. Serving size: about 2 cups. Preparation time: 10 minutes.

THE RECIPES: Condiments & Extras

The condiments in this section are further testimony to the importance of real food, balanced menus, and your eating satisfaction. These salad dressings, pestos, pâtés, sauces and spreads add eye appeal and delicious, mouth-watering flavor to your dishes. They are also specially designed to provide balanced nutrition, such as protein and essential fatty acids from nuts, seeds, and olives.

These condiments and extras are also designed with versatility and convenience in mind. You'll find basic condiment recipes with easy variations, and a number of classic sauces you can create by just adding an ingredient or two to the original basic recipe. Finally, in other recipes in this book, many of these condiments are included as ingredients, so you can instantly turn a plain broiled chicken or poached fish into an elegant entrée fit for dinner parties.

Asian Dressing

This zesty, piquant dressing can be used for salads, vegetable pasta, meat marinade, or dipping sauce.

³⁄₄	cup raw sesame seed tahini, almond or peanut butter
³⁄₄	cup brewed black tea
1	Tbsp apple juice
1	small chili pepper or ¹⁄₄ tsp chili flakes
2	cloves garlic, chopped
2	Tbsp tamari soy sauce
2	Tbsp fresh ginger, minced

Nutrition Facts

calories	total fat	carbs	protein
72	6g	3g	2g

1 place nut butter, tea, apple juice, chili, garlic, tamari, and ginger in blender container. Cover and blend on high until smooth.

2 dilute to desired consistency. Store in covered container in refrigerator.

Serves 16. Serving Size: 1 Tbsp per serving. Preparation time: 5 minutes.

Basic Herb Vinaigrette

This is a basic salad dressing you can vary with different herbs and seasonings.

¼	cup fresh lemon juice
¼	cup red wine or apple cider vinegar
⅓	cup extra virgin olive oil
3	med garlic cloves
3	Tbsp fresh parsley, basil or thyme leaves
2	med scallions or green onions
1	Tbsp Dijon Mustard
½	tsp Spike or Mrs. Dash vegetable seasoning
2	tsp apple juice

Nutrition Facts

calories	total fat	carbs	protein
58	3g	1g	0g

1 place all ingredients in blender container. Cover and process on high until blended.

2 transfer to glass jar with lid. Refrigerate at least ½ hour before serving, if possible. Keeps for several weeks.

Serves 12. Serving Size: 1 Tbsp per serving. Preparation time: 5 minutes.

variations

Sunny Seed Salad Dressing

add 2 Tbsp Savory Sunny Seed Mix and 2 tsp tamari soy sauce. Blend in food processor or blender until smooth.

Tomato Vinaigrette

add 2 tsp tomato paste to Basic Herb Vinaigrette and stir to blend.

Basic Mayonnaise Plus

This basic mayonnaise recipe can be varied to create many different sauces, including anchovy, garlic and curry mayos, remoulade, creamy Dijonnaise and tartar sauce.

2	egg yolks
1	tsp Dijon mustard
1	Tbsp lemon juice
1/2	tsp salt
	dash cayenne pepper
2/3	cup olive oil
1	oz firm silken tofu

1 in blender or food processor, place egg yolks, mustard, lemon juice, salt, and cayenne pepper.

2 blend momentarily to mix ingredients. Then with machine running, drizzle a thin, but steady stream of olive oil through hole in top, blending until mayonnaise thickens.

3 add tofu and blend. Check consistency. Remove to covered jar. Refrigerate.

4 if mayonnaise is too thick, blend in 1–2 teaspoons of hot water. This recipe can easily be made by hand in a small bowl with a wire whisk. The key is to gradually add the oil to the other ingredients in a thin, steady stream.

Serves 16. Serving size: 1 Tbsp per serving. Preparation time: 5 minutes.

Nutrition Facts

calories	total fat	carbs	protein
88	10g	0g	0g

remoulade variations

Remoulade

to 1 cup of Basic Mayonnaise, add 2 tsp capers, 1 tsp minced scallion or green onion, and 1 tsp minced parsley.

Dijon Remoulade

to 1 cup of Remoulade, add 2 Tbsp Dijon mustard.

Tartar Sauce

to 1 cup Remoulade, add 2 tsp dillweed and 1 Tbsp chopped dill pickles.

mayonnaise variations

Aioli Garlic Mayonnaise

to 1 cup of Basic Mayonnaise, add 1 Tbsp finely minced garlic. Blend until smooth.

Anchovy Mayonnaise

to 1 cup of Basic Mayonnaise, add 2 anchovy fillets, smashed.

Curry Mayonnaise

to 1 cup of Basic Mayonnaise, add 1/3 tsp curry powder.

Dijonnaise

to 1 cup of Basic Mayonnaise, add 2 Tbsp Dijon mustard.

Basil Pesto

The French classic pesto or "paste" of pine nuts, garlic, and herbs can also be made with walnuts, macadamia or other nuts, producing intense flavor and nutritional benefits in one potent spoonful.

2	cups fresh basil leaves, stemmed and packed
³⁄₄	cup fresh Italian flat-leaf parsley, chopped
¹⁄₂	cup walnuts
2	med garlic cloves
3	drops lemon oil or ¹⁄₂ tsp grated lemon rind (no white)
¹⁄₂	cup extra virgin olive oil
1	tsp sea salt
¹⁄₄	cup grated Parmesan or Romano cheese

1 in food processor workbowl combine all ingredients.

2 process until blended and fairly smooth. Store in covered container in refrigerator for up to 3 weeks.

Serves 24. Serving Size: 1 Tbsp per serving. Preparation time: 5 minutes.

Nutrition Facts

calories	total fat	carbs	protein
62	6g	1g	1g

Notes and Suggestions

Substitute high omega-3 fatty acid nuts like walnuts for pine nuts for a nutritonal, as well as flavor boost.

Black Olive Tapenade

This rich, hearty "pesto" can be pulled from the fridge for instant flavor, nutrition and gourmet elegance in appetizers, vegetables, dressings, snacks, meats and mains.

Nutrition Facts

calories	total fat	carbs	protein
61	4g	6g	1g

3/4	cup black olives, pitted
6	Tbsp walnuts (between 1/3 & 1/2 cup)
2	med garlic clove, smashed
1	small shallot or scallions, white only
1	cup spinach leaves, stemmed, chopped and packed
1/2	cup flat-leaf Italian parsley, stemmed, chopped and packed
1/4	cup fresh thyme leaves
3–4	drops lemon essential oil or 1/2 tsp grated lemon peel
1/2	tsp sea salt
3	Tbsp extra virgin olive oil

1 in food processor fitted with steel blade, combine nuts and garlic, process until ground. Add shallot or scallion, spinach, parsley, thyme leaves and salt. Process until ingredients are chunky and start to come together, 1–2 minutes.

2 add olive and lemon oils and process until mixture becomes a paste, but not smooth. Transfer to covered glass jar. Refrigerate for several weeks. Serve as dip, spread, snack or topping.

3 notes: Fresh herbs are definitely preferred, but 2 Tbsp dried thyme leaves can be substituted for fresh, if mixture stands before serving, so flavors can meld. Traditional pestos are usually made with Parmesan cheese, but lemon oil can give a tangy flavor boost without the dairy.

Serves 24. Serving Size: 1 Tbsp per serving. Preparation time: 10 minutes.

Chunky Mockamole

This amazingly authentic version of guacamole uses chopped vegetables to lower the calories.

2	cups asparagus cuts
2	med garlic cloves
2	med whole green onions, chopped
1	large celery stalk and leaves, finely chopped
1	serrano or chili pepper, seeded and minced
2	med ripe Haas avocados, peeled, pitted, and chunked (reserve whole avocado pits)
1	small tomato, seeded and chopped
¼	cup chopped cilantro
2	Tbsp fresh lemon or lime juice
½	tsp Spike vegetable seasoning or Mrs. Dash

Nutrition Facts

calories	total fat	carbs	protein
43	3g	3g	1g

Notes and Suggestions

Use this healthier version of guacamole as dip, fajita topping or Roll-Up filling.

1 steam asparagus pieces in a basket steamer or small amount of water for 3–4 minutes. Remove from heat, drain and place in large mixing bowl. Let cool to room temperature.

2 meanwhile, in food processor workbowl, combine garlic, onions, celery, and serrano pepper. Process with short bursts until vegetables are finely chopped.

3 smash steamed asparagus with the back of a spoon or pestle (from mortar and pestle) until still chunky. Add avocado chunks and mash mixture a bit more, but do not make it mushy.

4 add chopped vegetables, chopped tomato, cilantro, lemon juice, and Spike. Stir to mix. Cover tightly with waxed paper or plastic wrap and refrigerate for at least 20–30 minutes to let flavors develop. Add whole avocado pits to the Mockamole for increased preservation. Remove before serving.

5 if there is any Mockamole left, store tightly covered in refrigerator. Holds for one day.

Serves 16. Serving Size: 2 Tbsp per serving. Preparation time: 10 minutes.

Cornell BBQ Sauce

Without a doubt, the best non-tomato barbecue sauce going. Savory, piquant and pungent, but not spicy or sweet. No wonder it's been popular for almost 50 years!

1	cup coconut oil
2	cups cider vinegar
3	Tbsp salt
2	Tbsp poultry seasoning
½	tsp pepper
1	egg

Nutrition Facts

calories	total fat	carbs	protein
43	5g	1g	0g

Notes and Suggestions

The family will suddenly appear in the kitchen, noses sniffing the air when this vinegary sauce is simmering on the stove. This unique, piquant sauce is its outstanding best on BBQ chicken marinated and then cooked over a charcoal or gas grill. You can use it as a marinade for chicken or turkey done in the oven, it just won't be as outstanding. Recipe courtesy Cornell Co-operative Extension.

1 in heavy saucepan, combine oil, vinegar, salt, poultry seasoning, and pepper.

2 bring just up to the boiling point, reduce heat and simmer for 5–7 minutes. Remove from heat. For a thicker sauce, quickly whisk in beaten egg. Let cool.

3 store extra sauce, not used for BBQ, in glass jar with lid in refrigerator. Keeps for up to two months.

Serves 48. Serving Size: 1 Tbsp per serving. Preparation time: 10 minutes.

Green Olive Tomatillo Salsa

Roasting the tomatillos first adds a unique smoky flavor to this out-of-the-ordinary green olive salsa.

3	med tomatillos
2	med green tomatoes, finely chopped
1	serrano pepper, seeded and diced
2	med garlic cloves, minced
1/2	cup chopped red onion
1	Tbsp extra virgin olive oil
2	tsp sea salt
5–6	grinds freshly ground black pepper
1	Tbsp lime juice
2/3	cup green olives, chopped
1/4	cup chopped cilantro

Nutrition Facts

calories	total fat	carbs	protein
23	2g	2g	0g

1 remove husks and slice tomatillos lengthwise into 1/4" slices. Dry roast in heavy skillet or broil until brown, turning once. Remove from heat. Cool.

2 coarsely chop green tomatoes and add to skillet with pepper, garlic, onions, and olive oil. Sauté gently for 3–4 minutes, until tomatoes start to soften. Remove from heat.

3 into food processor workbowl, add roasted tomatillos and green tomato mixture, salt, pepper, lemon or lime juice, and green olives. Process until salsa is blended and chunky.

4 cilantro can be blended in at this point, if serving right away, However, flavor is much better if mixture is refrigerated for at least 1 hour (or up to 2 days) for flavors to meld. Blend chopped cilantro into salsa just before serving.

Serves 16. Serving Size: 1 Tbsp per serving. Preparation time: 10 minutes.

Miso Walnut Paste

A basic ingredient in oriental cooking, miso is a salty, fermented, soybean paste that plays a big role in adding flavor, depth, body, and nutrition to a wide variety of foods.

1	cup raw, organic walnuts
1	tsp rosemary leaves, crushed
2	Tbsp dark miso, fermented soybean paste

Nutrition Facts

calories	total fat	carbs	protein
53	5g	2g	1g

Notes and Suggestions

This spread can be used with vegetables, salads, snacks, appetizers, sprout and grated vegetable sandwich fillings, as a hearty protein and/or flavor topper for steamed vegetables, as a base for vegetarian paté blended with sautéed mushrooms, or as a savory crust for meats or fish.

1 lightly toast walnuts on cookie sheet in preheated 375°F. oven for 4–5 minutes.

2 in workbowl of food processor, add rosemary leaves while machine is running. Add hot nuts to food processor. Then add miso paste, processing until smooth and blended.

3 remove to glass container with tight fitting lid. Refrigerate for up to 6 weeks.

Serves 16. Serving size: 1 Tbsp per serving. Preparation time: 10 minutes.

Red Onion Cilantro Relish

This is a quick homemade salsa to add intense flavor, color and nutrition to plain protein or vegetable foods.

1	tsp extra virgin olive oil
1	med red onion, peeled and diced
1	tsp ginger root, minced
1	med garlic clove, minced
3	Tbsp fresh lemon juice
½	cup chopped fresh cilantro
¼	cup chopped fresh curly parsley
2	tsp capers

Nutrition Facts

calories	total fat	carbs	protein
5	0g	1g	0g

1 classically, the way to prepare this relish is to sauté onions in a small pan in olive oil until translucent, then add ginger and garlic, cooking for 30 seconds. Add lemon juice and heat until most of liquid has evaporated. Add remaining ingredients and cool.

2 practically and healthwise, the easiest and most nutritious way to prepare this salsa is with a food processor. Add all ingredients as listed, cover and pulse several times until relish ingredients are about equal size and blended. Do not overprocess.

3 serve as garnish or condiment on meat, fish, poultry, vegetables, salads.

Serves 24. Serving Size: 1 Tbsp per serving. Preparation time: 5 minutes.

Sea Salad Side

Once you try this unusual looking, nutrient-dense vegetable, it could become a favorite.

1	cup dry arame or hiziki seaweed
2	cups filtered water
1	med organic carrot, sliced into matchsticks
2	cloves garlic, sliced
1	med onion, crescent-sliced
1	Tbsp sesame oil
2	tsp tamari soy sauce

Nutrition Facts

calories	total fat	carbs	protein
64	4g	8g	1g

Notes and Suggestions

Serve this tasty, nutrient-rich, seaweed salad as a vegetable condiment to add color, flavor and nutrition to salads like Sea Salad, or to spark up a dinner plate.

1 pour water over dry seaweed in bowl. Set aside to rehydrate.

2 while seaweed is soaking, cut carrot into slices, then into matchsticks.

3 heat medium skillet, sauté garlic and onion in oil and tamari 1–2 minutes, then add carrots and sauté until carrot sticks start to soften, 2 minutes.

4 while sautéing, drain seaweed, reserving soaking liquid. Add rehydrated seaweed to skillet. Sauté lightly to absorb flavors. Add reserved soaking liquid. Simmer, covered, for 8–9 minutes.

5 remove from heat. Let cool slightly. Store in covered glass container in refrigerator up to 1 week.

Serves 4. Serving Size: $^1/4$ cup. Preparation time: 15 minutes.

Vegetable Essences

These magical, nutritious elixirs are intensely-flavored, brilliantly-colored infusions of vegetables and herbs, meant to be drizzled in tiny quantities over the finished plate.

Carrot Essence

Juice 4 large, organic carrots, about 1$\frac{1}{2}$ cups. Transfer to small saucepan and simmer very gently over medium low heat until juice has reduced to $\frac{1}{2}$ cup.

Blend with 1 garlic clove, 2 tsp lemon juice, 3–4 drops lemon oil or zest of $\frac{1}{2}$ lemon, and 1$\frac{1}{2}$ cups olive oil in blender or food processor until smooth. Transfer to squeeze bottle.

Parsley Essence

Blend 2 cups chopped, stemmed flat-leaf parsley with $\frac{1}{2}$ tsp salt, $\frac{1}{2}$ shallot, and 1 cup olive oil in food processor or blender. Transfer to squeeze bottle. Refrigerate. Drizzle over vegetables, salad, or as edible saucy garnish over serving plate.

Beet Essence

Juice 4 large beets in juice extractor, yielding about 1$\frac{1}{2}$ cups juice. Transfer to small saucepan and simmer gently over medium low heat until juice is reduced to $\frac{1}{2}$ cup.

Remove from heat and cool. Blend beet reduction with $\frac{1}{2}$ tsp salt, $\frac{1}{8}$ tsp cloves, several grinds of freshly ground black pepper, and 1$\frac{1}{2}$ cups olive oil in blender or food processor until smooth. Transfer to squeeze bottle and refrigerate.

Serving Size: $\frac{1}{8}$–$\frac{1}{2}$ tsp drizzle per serving. Preparation time: 30 minutes

Notes and Suggestions

Used by only a few select, high-end chefs, these brilliantly colored oils can add a bright burst of color, flavor, and nutrition as a garnish, especially for calorie and fat conscious CT's. Drizzle tiny quantities in a decorative crosshatch or swirl pattern over the finished plate. Simply prepare them during a batch session to have on hand for adding interest to a plate or dish that might otherwise call for higher fat/calorie cheese or nuts. These will keep for about two months in tightly covered squeeze bottles or jars in your refrigerator.

Appendix

Recommended Ingredients and Products Locator

Most of the foods used in this book's recipes, and the foods and health products recommended in Part One, can be found in health food stores or grocery stores. If you can't find them there, though, or if you want further insight on the best forms and brands of these foods and products, you can consult these lists below.

The first list contains all the foods and other health products and services that I have researched extensively, that are typically more difficult to find in stores, and that I offer through the "Recommended Products" section of Mercola.com. Some of these will be shipped directly from our own fulfillment center while others will be shipped to you directly from the farms and other suppliers.

The second list contains some specific foods and kitchen equipment that you can order direct from the suppliers or other online stores.

"Recommended Products" on Mercola.com

Beef, Grass-fed
100% Grass-fed beef high in CLA and omega-3 and containing no antibiotics or steroids.

Bison, Grass-fed and O.U. Certified Kosher
Many people call bison the most delicious of all red meats, and it also happens to be among the healthiest. This grass-fed bison, from the premier provider, Blackwing, is also certified as kosher, meaning you are getting the cleanest and healthiest meat available anywhere. Over 30 different cuts of this wildly popular meat are now available through Mercola.com.

Blueberry and Cherry Concentrate Softgel Capsules
Blueberries and cherries are densely packed with a variety of potent phytochemcials that normalize and improve health. These "CherryFlex" and "Wild Blueberry IQ" softgels taste great while maintaining the health benefits of whole fruit just as Mother Nature intended with a highly condensed serving of fresh fruit in a convenient once-a-day soft gel capsule. These non-pasteurized softgels are produced and tested to provide more disease fighting anthocyanins per serving than most competitors have in an entire bottle!

Cheese, Grass-fed Organic and Raw Milk

Brick, cheddar, feta, garlic & herb, mozzarella and two varieties of raw milk cheese, all from cows naturally pasture-raised on certified organic grasses. High in omega-3, CLA, and considerably higher in vitamins A, D and E than regular store-bought cheese.

Chicken, Free-Range Organic

Chicken raised on a 100% organic diet, no antibiotics or hormones, and in free-range conditions, means the healthiest, juiciest, most tender and delicious chicken you've ever tried. Our site offers whole chickens, boneless breasts, and thighs.

Chlorella

The highest quality and purest chlorella available, produced by Yaeyama, this natural food supplement is superior in total nutritional value to any man-made vitamin. High in many of the essential vitamins, minerals and enzymes—including all eight essential amino acids—and many micronutrients, chlorella will help build your immune system, detoxify the heavy metals and pesticides in your body, improve your digestive system, increase your energy and mental concentration, balance your body's pH, and much more.

Clenzology Advanced Hygiene System

Proper hygiene is critical to achieving and maintaining optimal health. We now know that germs aren't spread to us through coughing or sneezing as relatively few germs even become airborne, and fewer still actually bother us. In fact, they're handed to us during routine and intimate physical contact. The simple 5–step Clenzology process takes just minutes a day to perform and focuses on cleaning the areas of your body that most dramatically affect the overall quality of your health—your hands, face, ears, mouth, and nose.

CocoChia—The Ultimate Snack Fuel

A blend of the finest organic shredded coconut and whole organic chia seeds, CocoChia is antimicrobial, helpful for fatigue and weight loss, and absolutely delicious! Plus, this "ultimate snack food" is loaded with essential vitamins, fatty acids, and antioxidants.

Coconut Oil, Virgin and Organic

Virgin coconut oil is highly recommended for your cooking, and has a wide range of proven health benefits. But quality can vary widely among brands, so you have to know what you are looking for. Tropical Traditions and Garden of Life brand coconut oils meet all the necessary requirements, including certified organic, non-GMO, no "copra" or dried coconuts used, and no hydrogenation.

Fish Oil and Cod Liver Oil

Fish oil and cod liver oil are among the few supplements (though they really are a food) that everyone should take, as they are ideal sources of omega-3 with DHA and EPA fatty acids that are dangerously lacking in most people's diets. There is great variance in quality among brands, though: three brands I highly recommend are the Garden of Life Olde World Icelandic cod liver oil, the Living Fuel Omega-3 & E capsules (with full-spectrum vitamin E included!) and the Carlson's brand of fish oil, all available here.

Juicer, Omega 8002 Model

I have done an extensive evaluation of juicers and found that the Omega 8002 Juicer is the clear winner in terms of its multiple uses, durability, ease of use and cleaning, and value. You can find an extensive juicer evaluation chart comparing the various juicers here as well.

Kefir Starter and Culture Starter

Traditionally fermented foods are an essential part of every healthy diet, and the Kefir Starter and Culture Starter available here an exceptionally high-quality way to make your own fermented foods very quickly and inexpensively. Kefir is an ancient—and still one of nature's most powerful and delicious—health foods, and the Kefir Starter enables very easy preparation. The Culture Starter, meanwhile, is a simple way to make your vegetables into very healthy and delicious traditional fermented foods.

Living Fuel Rx "Superfood"

I have extensively researched quick and convenient foods claiming to be healthy, and this is the only one I highly recommend. It is exceptional as a healthy meal replacement or to supplement your daily nutrition, as it provides complete and natural concentrated sources of vitamins, minerals, proteins, essential fats, enzymes and co-enzymes, and plant fibers. It is available in both a greens and berry variety.

Ostrich, Free-Range

Ostrich is an exceptionally healthy red meat that tastes like chicken, but is lower in fat, calories and cholesterol than even skinless chicken or turkey. It can be used in place of virtually any meat, such as beef, chicken or pork, in your favorite recipes, and is even available in an omega-3-rich variety.

Raw Milk & Raw Dairy Products

Through Mercola.com you now have access to raw milk, butter and cream from the one existing source of "real" organic raw dairy that can ship anywhere in the U.S! The unique pasture-based mobile dairy produces milk naturally low in bacteria. The cows graze on green pastures all year long and never return to manure-filled pens for milking. Never processed, never pasteurized and never homogenized, these raw dairy products are high in antioxidants, vitamins (including B-12), all 22 essential amino acids, natural enzymes, natural probiotics and good fatty acids. None of the cows are ever given antibiotics, hormones or GMOs.

Salmon, Wild Red Alaskan and Toxin-Free

This Vital Choice brand of salmon is the only fish I have found, through independent laboratory testing we had performed on the fish, to be free from harmful mercury, PCBs and other toxins. It is a premier source of omega-3 with EHA and DPA fatty acids, is high in antioxidants, and is free of antibiotics, pesticides, synthetic coloring agents, growth hormones and GMOs. It also tastes absolutely incredible!

Sun Alarm Clock by Soleil

Sunlight is an essential element in staying healthy. Now you can reap the benefits of waking up naturally with the Sun Alarm Clock. You'll wake up the way nature intended, giving you more energy for the day ahead. Combining the features of a traditional alarm clock (digital display, AM/FM radio, beeper, snooze button, etc) with a special built-in light that gradually increases in intensity, simulating a natural sunrise. Included is a sunset feature where the light fades to darkness over time—ideal for kids or anyone who has trouble falling asleep. Plus, if you are a very sound sleeper this alarm will flash and beep at the end of the alarm cycle to assist you with waking.

Vitamin D

Most people do not get enough sunlight—the best source of vitamin D—and are therefore deficient in this crucial vitamin. I highly recommend you get tested for your vitamin D levels, and if you are deficient, strongly encourage you to first read Richard Hobday's remarkable book, *The Healing Sun* (see "Recommended Books" below.) Learn how to get the proper amount of sun exposure—a free, enjoyable and very necessary health "supplement"—and if you need to further supplement with vitamin D, I encourage you to use a pure, high-quality supplement like Living Fuel's D&A.

Vitamin K

Proven to help build your bones and help your heart, most people do not get enough vitamin K from their daily diet and should consider supplementing it. This is a full five-month supply of the natural vitamin K I highly recommend, available at an excellent price.

Water Evaluation and Home Water Testing

Clean and healthy tap water, whether provided by your municipality or a well, is essential for your health whether you cook, clean, or bathe with it. You can get an instant free evaluation of your municipality's water supply here, and a range of discounted EPA-certified home water tests.

Foods—Other Suppliers

Almond Flour
Grain-free thickener or flour
Bob's Red Mill Natural Foods, 1-800-349-2173, www.bobsredmill.com

Arrowroot Flour
Grain-free thickener or flour
Frontier Natural Products, 1-800-669-3275, www.frontiercoop.com

Bean Flour
Low-carb bean flour mixes
Kitchen ET Cetera, Inc., 1-877-655-1415, www.beanflour.com

Full-fat Soy Flour
Available in most health food stores. Note: I am not a big advocate of unfermented soy products. Nevertheless, soy flour is found in most health food stores, is low in carbohydrates, and can be used in occasional tablespoon doses.

Herbs and Seasonings, Organic
Frontier Natural Products, 1-800-669-3275, www.frontiercoop.com

Milk and Cream, Raw
Go to www.realmilk.com to find out if there are cow-share programs in your area
Nuts and Seeds, Raw and Organic
Jaffe Brothers Natural Foods, 1-760-749-1133, www.organicfruitsandnuts.com

Psyllium Seeds and Husks
Frontier Natural Products (*see* Arrowroot Flour)
Bob's Red Mill Natural Foods (*see* Almond Flour)

Spike®/Salt-Free Spike
Famous all-purpose vegetable seasoning
Modern Products, 1-800-877-8935, www.modernfearn.com or in most grocery stores

Sprouting Seeds, Organic
Complete line of organic seeds
The Sproutpeople, 1-877-777-6887, www.sproutpeople.com

Stevia
Non-carb, non-glycemic, non-synthetic, alternative sweetener
Available in liquid concentrate and baking powder
Body Ecology, 1-800-511-2660, bodyecologydiet.com

Tahini
Raw, hulled & unhulled organic sesame paste
Oskri Organics, 1-800-628-1110, www.oskri.com

Whey Powder
Dairy by-product that aids digestion, natural culturing
Frontier Natural Products (*see* Arrowroot Flour)
Bob's Red Mill Natural Foods (*see* Almond Flour)

Kitchen Equipment—Other Suppliers

Food Dehydrators
Excalibur Dehydrator®
Excalibur Products, 1-800-875-4254, www.excaliburdehydrator.com

Juicers
See "Juicer, Omega 8002 Model," under "Recommended Products on Mercola.com"

Spiral Slicer™
Manual slicer & processor for creating pasta from vegetables
Joyce Chen Products, 1-800-333-0208, www.joycechen.com

Sprouters
Sprouting equipment and seeds
The Sproutpeople, 1-877-777-6887, www.sproutpeople.com

Recommended Resources and Further Reading

Books
These highly recommended books and more, including full and original reviews, are available through the "Recommended Products" section of Mercola.com. Most are also available at bookstores and your local library. When you purchase them through Mercola.com, you will get them at the lowest prices at Amazon.com, BN.com or other online stores. Mercola.com receives a small percentage of each of these sales that goes toward both being able to keep the "eHealthy News You Can Use" e-newsletter described below free, and toward expanding all the other free offerings on the site.

The Cholesterol Myths: Exposing the Fallacy that Saturated Fat and Cholesterol Cause Heart Disease
Dr. Uffe Ravnskov
Dr. Ravnskov is the author of numerous articles published in major medical journals. This book elaborates on the lack of connection between diet, blood cholesterol levels and heart disease and questions the widespread use of cholesterol-lowering drugs. Physicians and other health professionals, as well as those facing cholesterol-lowering treatments, would be both enlightened and better able to resist worthless treatments by reading this book.

The Fluoride Deception
Christopher Bryson
If you've ever read that warning on the back of your toothpaste tube—the one that says a child who swallows more than a pea-size amount should contact poison control—and won-

dered how fluoridated water, which people drink in uncontrolled quantities, could be safe in comparison, do not miss this book. Author Christopher Bryson cites numerous scientific studies linking fluoride to numerous health ills including arthritis, bone cancer, emphysema and nervous system disorders like Alzheimer's disease and attention deficit disorder (ADD).

Getting Things Done
David Allen

This is one of the most useful and important books I have ever read. If you are challenged in any way with organizing your life, making plans, and sticking to those plans, you should read this brilliant book. It provides practical, realistic, hands-on and time-tested insight on greatly improving your productivity, including a full slate of tips, tools and techniques.

Having a Baby, Naturally
Peggy O'Mara

If you are an expectant parent, or know someone who is, this is an exceptional book by the editor and publisher of Mothering magazine that provides comprehensive insight on how to ensure the health of your baby, and the health of the expectant mother, including diet and exercise, emotional self-awareness, birth choices and locations, breastfeeding, and more.

The Healing Sun
Richard Hobday

Richard Hobday has created a remarkable book to help us understand the true value of proper sun exposure. Most people no longer realize that we require regular exposure to sunshine to optimize our health. In fact, many people are dangerously deficient in vitamin D, and the sun is by far the best source of obtaining the required vitamin D. Unfortunately over the last 40 years, the medical community has pushed the concerns with excessive UV rays to such extremes that people now believe they have to avoid the sun, which can have very dire consequences. This is one of the most important books I have read in recent years, and if you are "scared of the sun" I urge you to move this book to the top of your reading list so you can avoid some potentially very serious health issues.

Healing Words
Larry Dossey

A classic work on the proven link between spirituality and health by a leading physician. Provides both documented evidence and real-life examples to show that prayer and spirituality can indeed be a valid healing tool. A compelling read no matter what your religious/spiritual background.

How to Eat, Move and Be Healthy!
Paul Chek
This beautifully written and detailed book provides a complete plan—from proper diet through sensible exercise—that is easy to understand and fully realistic for anyone to implement in their lives. This book is, in fact, a perfect complement to the book you are holding in your hands now, as the two work synergistically to provide everything you need to know to improve your health and wellness, including Chek's complete step-by-step guide showing you how to create your individual exercise plan.

Impossible Cure: The Promise of Homeopathy
Amy Lansky, Ph.D.
Amy Lansky, former NASA researcher with a Standord Ph.D., tells the incredible story of how she used homeopathy to cure her son of autism. In this compelling and easy to understand description of how homeopathy can be used to treat "incurable conditions" like autism, Lansky also provides an in-depth account on the history, philosophy and practice of homeopathy, as well as dozens of other testimonials on the power of homeopathy in curing various health problems.

Know Your Fats: Complete Primer for Understanding the Nutrition of Fats, Oils and Cholesterol
Mary G. Enig, Ph.D.
This book, by a leading dietary fat and oil researcher, dispels the myths about saturated fat and oils previously thought of as unhealthy, and pinpoints those that truly are. It also provides an in-depth guide to the critical relationship between dietary fat intake and health and disease prevention. Written broad enough to appeal to the general public, but with sufficient detail to serve as an excellent reference to medical practitioners as well.

Living Well with Hypothyroidism: What Your Doctor Doesn't Tell You, What You Need to Know
Mary J. Shomon
If you are challenged by hypothyroidism, or suspect you may be, this book is one of the most insightful, unbiased and useful resources you can read on the subject. Mary Shomon is a nationally respected thyroid expert who presents her information in a highly readable format.

The Makers Diet
By Jordan S. Rubin, N.M.D., Ph.D.
Rubin's program is designed around attacking the "Three I's" that have everything to do with the chronic diseases that are currently plaguing the nation: insulin, infection, and inflammation. Rubin then provides a full range of very sound solutions that are holistic in the truest sense of the word, incorporating the physical, spiritual, mental and emotional on the roadmap to your health and well-being.

The Metabolic Typing Diet: Customize Your Diet to Your Own Unique Body Chemistry
William L. Wolcott, with Trish Fahey
After reading the book you now hold in your hands, this book, by the leading metabolic typing expert of our time, is an ideal follow-up. It provides a full understanding of metabolic typing and offers extensive and highly practical information on how to fine-tune your diet for your specific biochemistry. It also provides a more comprehensive test to determine your metabolic type (if, via the metabolic test in this book, you determined that you are a Mixed Type, I strongly urge you to take the test in Wolcott's book, as it will provide a more succinct answer to your type.)

The No-Grain Diet
Dr. Joseph Mercola, with Alison Rose Levy
My previous book, a New York Times bestseller, provides an easy-to-follow three-phase program that is particularly useful for those trying to lose weight. While The No-Grain Diet doesn't contain the detailed insight on metabolic typing, many overweight and obese people have found great success with the plan presented in this book. It also provides detailed insight on how to learn and use EFT, a remarkably effective emotional healing tool.

Nutrition and Physical Degeneration
Dr. Weston Price
I often my refer patients to this wonderful resource. This is a pioneering work in natural health and simply a must-read if you are interested in natural medicine in any way. Dr. Westin Price was one of the most prominent dentists at the turn of the century and wondered why so many children were getting cavities. He realized that it was the introduction of processed foods. So he traveled the world and documented the connection between processed foods and ill health, and the principles he developed still largely hold true today.

The Omega-3 Connection:
The Groundbreaking Anti-Depression Diet and Brain Program
Andrew L. Stoll, M.D.
Dr. Stoll is a psychiatrist from Harvard and his book does an outstanding and thorough job detailing the strong connection between fish oils high in omega-3 and depression. If you or someone you love suffers from depression, this book provides a real solution and is a must-read.

Our Toxic World: A Wake-Up Call
Dr. Doris Rapp
Everyday we are exposed to numerous chemicals, many of which we're not even aware, that wreak havoc upon our health. These chemicals saturate our environment from the air we breathe to the water we drink. They're in the homes we live in and the products we use, and all of us are at risk. Dr. Doris Rapp, board certified in environmental medicine, pediatrics and allergy, has written this book that is truly the wake-up call we need on this important topic.

The Paleo Diet
Loren Cordain, Ph.D.
Dr. Cordain is considered one of the world's leading experts on Paleolithic nutrition, and his ideas have definitely had a strong influence on my dietary program. This book is an easy to understand, authoritative reference on the scientific documentation for reducing our grain consumption to be more in line with our ancient ancestors.

The UV Advantage
Michael Holick, M.D., Ph.D.
This important book focuses on a crucial but little-known fact: the sun is one of your greatest allies when it comes to fighting disease, feeling great and living longer. "Your overall well-being depends in part on developing an appropriate relationship with the sun," says Dr. Michael Holick, M.D., one of the foremost authorities on vitamin D, a full Professor of medicine, dermatology, biophysics and physiology at the Boston University School of Medicine, and author of this groundbreaking book. If you've been hiding from the sun because of "expert" warnings to avoid it, find out the truth in this must-read book.

Virgin Coconut Oil:
How it Has Changed People's Lives, and How it Can Change Yours
Brian and Marianita Shilhavy
In this exceptional book you will learn why coconut oil is a true health "superfood" designed by God with exceptional antiviral, antibacterial and antifungal properties and the ability to considerably strengthen your immune system. You'll also learn how it can help you lose weight, prevent premature aging while rejuvenating your skin, improve conditions in those with diabetes, chronic fatigue, fibromyalgia, and much more.

The Whole Soy Story
Dr. Kaayla Daniel
This extensively researched and compelling read dispels the myths that soybeans are a major "health food" and pinpoints why they can lead to health challenges instead.

Your Body's Many Cries for Water
Dr. Fereydoon Batmanghelidj
This extensively researched and fascinating book demonstrates the strong connection between drinking clean and healthy water and fighting and preventing disease. The general public and health care practitioners alike would benefit immensely from reading this groundbreaking book.

Video and Audio Resources

Look for these video and audio health resources in the "Recommended Products" section of Mercola.com.

EFT Training Course
Gary Craig

EFT is profoundly effective emotional and mental healing approach that is based on the principles of energy medicine. I have taught it to the patients in my clinic for years, and they have experienced truly incredible and permanent results with it. If you have any type of emotional/mental issues that may be blocking your health and dietary success, I urge you to consider "The EFT Course" by Gary Craig, the pioneer of EFT that I also learned from. The EFT Course contains over 13 hours of video instruction (on DVD or VHS) on all the EFT basics as well as the "art of delivery," and comes with a 60-day money back guarantee.

Insight & Focus Audio CDs

The Insight audio CD is an exceptional tool to help you dramatically reduce the stress that is a prime contributor to all forms of disease while maximizing your awareness and potential for growth. The Focus 2–CD set is an extraordinary audio technology that will help you improve your levels of concentration and clarity, and increase your memory, creativity and problem-solving skills. From the moment you first listen to this audio technology, your brain will begin the process of reorganizing itself for higher thinking and enhanced levels of consciousness.

The Sedona Method Course—CD Program
Hale Dwoskin

As an alternative to EFT, many people have found "The Sedona Method" a highly effective emotional healing tool, and a tool to increase success and happiness. While The Sedona Method book is a good approach, this 13-CD audio program is easily the most effective way to learn this method, and also an incredible value.

Sweet Misery: A Poisoned World
Documentary on DVD

If you or anyone you love think aspartame is an accepticable dietary aid, this is true must-see TV! Long-term aspartame use can create a ticking time-bomb for a large array of neurological illnesses, including brain cancer, Lou Gehrig's Disease, Graves Disease, chronic fatigue, MS and epilepsy. "Sweet Misery" starts with filmmaker and narrator Cori Brackett's poignant story about how she discovered aspartame's ill effect on her health. Brackett's journey takes us across the United States to learn more about the devastating effects of aspartame from an impressive list of medical experts including Dr. Russell Blaylock, Dr. John Olney and Dr. Ralph G. Walton, to name a few. The film also features Arthur Evangelista, a former FDA investigator who exposes the medical horrors resulting from the use of aspartame in food and drinks.

This is one of the best DVDs I have seen on health and I highly recommend and endorse this movie. If you know someone who is using artificial sweeteners, share this movie with them—it could save their life!

Newsletters

In addition to my free e-newsletter listed below, there are a number of other excellent newsletters that provide insights you can really use in your journey to optimal health and wellness. This short list provides a representative sample.

Body Ecology Diet Updates

Subscribe at BodyEcologyDiet.com

This is a must-read e-newsletter focusing on dietary health and wellness, with a particular focus on the extreme importance of probiotics in your diet. If you are not yet completely aware of how crucial probiotics (and the naturally fermented foods they can be obtained from) are to your health—including your ability to avoid disease and look and feel younger —do not miss this newsletter from one of the world's leading authorities on probiotics, Donna Gates.

Dr. Mercola's "eHealthy News You Can Use"

Subscribe at www.Mercola.com

My free twice-weekly newsletter reaching 300,000 subscribers as of this writing, "eHealthy News You Can Use" provides you the most important and timely news and information that can really help you improve your health for good. I do not accept any third-party advertising and am not tied into any corporate or third party "special interests," so you get all the facts you really need to know, with insights provided by me and a team of the nation's leading health experts.

Bottom Line Health Newsletter

Subscribe at www.bottomlinesecrets.com

An outstanding health newsletter in both print and free e-newsletter format that provides easy-to-understand and worthwhile information geared toward consumers.

H.S.I. e-Alert

Subscribe at www.hsibaltimore.com

Another excellent e-newsletter providing news of urgent medical issues and health solutions, including breakthroughs in complementary and alternative medicine.

McAlvany Health Alert

Subscribe at www.mcalvanyhealthalert.com

This print newsletter, subtitled "The Journal of Healthy Aging," is an outstanding tool geared toward helping seniors in particular become and stay healthy in terms of body, mind and spirit.

Websites

www.Mercola.com

My website, with 30,000 pages of useful articles and information on virtually any health topic you are interested in, is now the world's most visited natural health website, and one of the world's six most visited health websites overall as of this writing. Whenever you have a question about any health or dietary topic, simply go to Mercola.com and enter the phrase in the powerful—and free—search engine. Also visit the "Find a Health Practitioner in Your Area" link at the bottom of the homepage for lists and contact information to EFT and other therapists.

www.bodyecologydiet.com

To improve your health in general, and especially if you have an immune disorder or candida-related imbalance, I strongly recommend you check out this website. Founder Donna Gates is renowned for her program's success in helping people overcome candidiasis and other immune-related disorders, and her program provides a particular focus on the powerful health benefits of fermented foods and probiotics that anyone seeking to be healthy should not miss.

www.eftupdate.com

For comprehensive insight on EFT, the "Emotional Freedom Technique," this is a highly useful and informative website. Founded and directed by Dr. Patricia Carrington, this site includes her own effective EFT learning courses.

www.emofree.com

For comprehensive insight on EFT, this is another highly useful and informative website, founded and directed by Gary Craig, the EFT pioneer. It also includes his highly effective EFT learning courses.

www.mothering.com

An excellent website for parents with a focus on natural approaches in terms of children's health and more.

www.realmilk.com

A fantastic resource by The Weston A. Price Foundation providing everything you need to know about healthy raw milk. Includes detail on why raw milk is so nutritious, if its sales are legal in your regions, and where specifically to find cowshare programs or suppliers in your area.

www.redflagsdaily.com

A compelling and expansive website that provides straightforward and unabashed insight on all the healthcare issues facing you today.

Fine-Tuning Your Diet to Your Metabolic Type Table

Make copies of the following table and use it to help you listen to your body after eating meals and fine-tune your diet, as explained in Chapter 5 and detailed throughout the recipes in this book.

FOOD INTAKE list all foods & drinks consumed			FINE TUNE YOUR DIET		
date:			please a check to the left of all descriptions that describe your experience 1–2 hours after each meal		
breakfast lunch dinner (circle one)	appetite satiety cravings		feel full, satisfied		feel physically full, but still hungry
			do NOT have sweet cravings		have desire for something sweet
			do NOT desire more food		feel physically full, but still hungry
			do NOT feel hungry		already hungry
foods consumed:			do NOT need to snack before next meal		feel need for a snack
	energy levels		energy feels renewed		meal gave too much or too little energy
			have good lasting "normal" sense of energy		became hyper, jittery, shaky, nervous or speedy
			energy tanked from meal- exhaustion, sleepiness, drowsiness, listlessness or lethargy		feel hyper but exhausted underneath
	mind / emotions / well-being		improved well-being		mentally slow
			sense of feeling refueled, renewed and restored		inability to think quickly or clearly
			some emotional upliftment		hyper, overly rapid thoughts
			improved mental clarity and sharpness		inability to focus or concentrate
			normalization of thought process		apathy, sadness, depression withdrawal
					anxious, fearful, angry or irritable

Reprinted with permission from The Metabolic Typing Diet: Customize Your Diet to Your Own Unique Body Chemistry *by William Wolcott, Doubleday Books, 2000*

Index of Recipes

Content Index

The Latest Health and Diet News that Can Truly Help You is Now Available Twice-Weekly—for FREE!

Go to www.Mercola.com. Enter your email address. Change your life.
That's all it takes to receive your twice-weekly copy of one of the world's most influential, discussed and useful health newsletters.

Do you want to take control of your health without letting it consume your entire life? Do you want all the latest health and dietary news that can really help you prevent disease, optimize weight, look and feel younger, and live longer—without having to spend your valuable time tracking it all down on your own? And you want all this for FREE?

Then simply go to Mercola.com and enter your email address to subscribe to Dr. Mercola's "eHealthy News You Can Use" e-newsletter. That's it. That's all. On a twice-weekly basis, you will now receive one of the world's most respected health and dietary sources filled with articles providing you crucial insights such as:

- Six steps you should take right now to have younger-looking skin
- The most successful secrets to losing weight and keeping it off permanently
- The five foods that provide a powerful boost to your intelligence
- Real solutions to end the pain from common illnesses and health disorders
- Why healthcare costs keep rising, but how you can save thousands of dollars
- How to overcome depression and feeling "down" once and for all
- The ten most toxic foods that you definitely should not eat
- What vitamins and supplements you really need, and those you don't
- The top foods that hold the real key to help you live longer
- The most dangerous pharmaceuticals to avoid, and real solutions that you can use to fight and prevent the underlying causes of disease instead
- How to find the best medical practitioners for you, from doctors to emotional therapists to chiropractors
- Six ways to prevent the flu and colds—and the flu shot isn't one of them
- The sugars and sugar substitutes you must avoid, and what you should use instead
- How to win the battle against specific diseases and health challenges, from diabetes, heart disease, and cancer to back pain, stomach problems and depression
- The five deadliest household tragedies, and how you can avoid them

You'll find insight like this and much more contributed by Dr. Mercola and a wide host of other leading health care experts in every free edition of "eHealthy News You Can Use." Plus, entirely free as well, you can use the powerful search feature on Mercola.com—now one of the world's most visited health websites with over 50,000 pages of information—to find real answers on any health and diet topic that matters to you.

So go to Mercola.com. Enter your email address. And change your life—for free.